OXFORD ASSESS AND PROGRESS

Psychiatry

Edited by

Gil Myers

Child and Adolescent Psychiatrist, Tavistock and Portman NHS
Foundation Trust
Honorary Clinical Teaching Fellow in Medical Education, University
College London Medical School

Melissa Gardner

General Practitioner, Killick Street Health Centre, London
Clinical Teaching Fellow, University College London Medical School

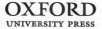

OXFORD
UNIVERSITY PRESS

OXFORD
UNIVERSITY PRESS

Great Clarendon Street, Oxford, OX2 6DP,
United Kingdom

Oxford University Press is a department of the University of Oxford.
It furthers the University's objective of excellence in research, scholarship,
and education by publishing worldwide. Oxford is a registered trade mark of
Oxford University Press in the UK and in certain other countries

First Edition published in 2014

Impression: 1

Published in the United States of America by Oxford University Press
198 Madison Avenue, New York, NY 10016, United States of America

British Library Cataloguing in Publication Data

Data available

Library of Congress Control Number: 2014931567

ISBN 978–0–19–966566–2

Printed in Great Britain by
Ashford Colour Press Ltd, Gosport, Hampshire

Series Editor Preface

The Oxford Assess and Progress Series is a groundbreaking development in the extensive area of self-assessment texts available for medical
students. The questions were specifically commissioned for the Series,
written by practising clinicians, extensively peer reviewed by students
and their teachers, and quality assured to ensure that the material is up
to date, accurate, and in line with modern testing formats.

The Series has a number of unique features and is designed as much
as a formative learning resource as a self-assessment one. The questions
are constructed to test the same clinical problem-solving skills that we
use as practising clinicians, rather than just testing theoretical knowledge,
namely:

- Gathering and using data required for clinical judgement
- Choosing examination, investigations, and interpretation of the findings
- Applying knowledge
- Demonstrating diagnostic skills
- Ability to evaluate undifferentiated material
- Ability to prioritize
- Making decisions and demonstrating a structured approach to deci-
  sion making

Each question is bedded in reality and typically is presented as a clinical
scenario, the contents of which have been chosen to reflect the common and important conditions that most doctors are likely to encounter
both during their training and in exams! The aim of the Series is to build
the reader's confidence around recognizing important symptoms and
signs and suggesting the most appropriate investigations and management and, in so doing, aid development of a clear approach to patient
management which can be transferred to the wards.

The content of the Series has deliberately been pinned to the relevant
Oxford Handbook but, in addition, has been guided by a blueprint that
reflects the themes identified in Tomorrow's Doctors and Good Medical
Practice to include novel areas such as history taking, recognition of signs
including red flags, and professionalism.

Particular attention has been paid to giving learning points and con-
structive feedback on each question, using clear fact- or evidence-based
explanations as to why the correct response is right and why the incorrect responses are less appropriate. The question editorials are clearly
referenced to the relevant sections of the accompanying Oxford
Handbook and/or more widely to medical literature or guidelines. They
are designed to guide and motivate the reader, being multipurpose in
nature, covering, for example, exam technique, approaches to difficult
subjects, and links between subjects.

Another unique aspect of the Series is the element of competency
progression from being a relatively inexperienced student to a more
experienced junior doctor. We have suggested the following four

degrees of difficulty to reflect the level of training so the reader can monitor their own progress over time, namely:

★   Graduate should know
★★   Graduate nice to know
★★★   Foundation should know
★★★★   Foundation nice to know

We advise the reader to attempt the questions in blocks as a way of testing knowledge in a clinical context. The Series can be treated as a dress rehearsal for life on the ward by using the material to hone clinical acumen and build confidence by encouraging a clear, consistent, and rational approach, proficiency in recognizing and evaluating symptoms and signs, making a rationale differential diagnosis, and suggesting appropriate investigations and management.

Adopting such an approach can aid not only being successful in examinations, which really are designed to confirm learning, but also, more importantly, being a good doctor. In this way we can deliver high quality and safe patient care by recognizing, understanding, and treating common problems, but at the same time remaining alert to the possibility of less likely but potentially catastrophic conditions.

David Sales and Katharine Boursicot

A Note on Single Best Answer and Extended Matching Questions

Single Best Answer questions are currently the format of choice being widely used by most undergraduate and postgraduate knowledge tests, and hence most of the assessment questions in this book follow this format.

Briefly, the Single Best Answer question presents a problem, usually a clinical scenario, before presenting the question itself and a list of five options. Of these five, there is one correct answer and four incorrect options or 'distractors' from which the reader chooses a response.

Extended Matching Questions are also known as extended matching items and were introduced as a more reliable way of testing knowledge. They are still currently widely used in many undergraduate and postgraduate knowledge tests, and hence are included in this book.

An Extended Matching Question is organized as one list of possible options followed by a set of items, usually clinical scenarios. The correct response to each item must be chosen from the list of options.

All of the questions in this book, which typically are based on an evaluation of symptoms, signs, or results of investigations either as single entities or in combination, are designed to test reasoning skills rather than straightforward recall of facts, and use cognitive processes similar to those used in clinical practice.

The peer-reviewed questions are written and edited in accordance with contemporary best assessment practice and their content has been guided by a blueprint pinned to all areas of Good Medical Practice, which ensures comprehensive coverage.

The answers and their rationales are evidence based and have been reviewed to ensure that they are absolutely correct. Incorrect options are selected as being plausible and indeed may look correct to the less knowledgeable reader. When answering questions, readers may wish to use the 'cover' test in which they read the scenario and the question but cover the options.

Preface

Psychiatry is fascinating. As a subject it rests in the interaction between biological, social, and psychological factors. While there is an underpinning of medical knowledge, diagnoses can alter with cultural and societal influences. Backed up by the latest research and by using innovative approaches to engage with a sometimes difficult to reach population, psychiatry can save lives and help people regain their confidence, worth, and place in the world. To do any of this, we need to have a genuine interest in people: what drives them, scares them, and makes them do what they do—for good and for bad. It is this curiosity in each other and how to solve these dilemmas that makes psychiatry as appealing to the trainee as to the skilled practitioner.

But that isn't why you will want to buy this book. The *Oxford Handbook of Psychiatry* is a brilliant gateway into the different approaches used to gain this knowledge. It offers an insightful look at the different parts of psychiatry and the historical influences that have made modern psychiatry such a rich specialty. We want to reflect this in the style of the book and hope that readers will be encouraged by the attention to higher learning rather than simply repeating back learned statements and rehearsed responses.

In medical education there has been a move toward expecting students to understand concepts rather than simply swallowing then regurgitating key facts to 'pass' one exam and move onto the next. Assessments are changing to reflect the shift in demand. True/False questions were easy to write but easy to get wrong in the exam, when a sneaky examiner stuck a 'not' in the lead, and therefore didn't differentiate between students. Now, there is a mix of Single Best Answer and Extended Matching Questions which aim to fairly test students about the important topics and allow them to plan and demonstrate their grasp of psychiatry. We want to help with that.

We believe that good questions test a fundamental, relevant point and provide a succinct, evidence-based answer to why the correct answer is correct and why wrong answers aren't. It's annoying spending time coming up with an answer only to find it isn't the one selected by the writer, or worse being told the answer is wrong but not *why* it's wrong. We want to explain our thinking. Single Best Answers use 'plausible distracters' to tempt the student into making an error, so these need to be clarified and the *best* answer justified. This is as true for the simple, common questions as it is for more complicated areas.

Our intention is to push learning forward by choosing essential testing points, providing explanations around these, and promoting further reading and understanding. It is our belief that by first understanding the basics, our readers will be persuaded to delve deeper into the subject—having already passed their exams with ease!

Gil Myers and Melissa Gardner

Acknowledgements

Thank you to all the chapter authors for their time and energy in creating questions that demonstrate such an interesting array of learning points. It was wonderful to see clinical expertise being used to generate fresh ideas and promote understanding through detailed explanation and shared experiences. For their valued feedback we would also like to thank the reviewers, both professional and student, who helped shape each question in the book through their thoughtful comment and considered responses.

On a personal note, we would like to mention a few people who shared their unique understanding of medical education, and in particular question writing, with us before, during, and continuing after the book has been published: Dr Alison Sturrock is an inspiring lead to the clinical teaching fellows at University College London Medical School (UCLMS) and Dr David Sales has a wealth of knowledge of all things to do with medical education. Thanks too to Dr Emily Titherington who took time out of her final year at medical school to help design the blueprint we used to develop the book chapters and advise us on content.

Finally, we would like to thank our families: Katie, Toby, Mel, and Rosalind (Gil) and Shaun, mom Katie, and Caroline (Melissa) for their continued support, both emotional and practical, and for their patience with the temporary disruption of our work–life balance during the writing of this book.

Acknowledgements

Contents

About the Editors

Volume Editors

Gil Myers is a child and adolescent psychiatrist working in North London. He trained at the Royal Free and the Maudsley Hospitals before completing a secondment at UCLMS. This involved developing fitness to practise assessments for the General Medical Council and undergraduate assessment of psychiatry and curricula development. He currently balances his clinical practice with continued work within the medical school, completing a master's degree in medical education at the Institute of Education, and caring for his young daughter.

Melissa Gardner is a salaried General Practitioner in King's Cross, London, and a clinical teaching fellow at UCLMS. She graduated from UCLMS in 2006, and completed the Whittington VTS scheme in 2011. She is enjoying combining her interest in medical education with her clinical work and has particular interests in community-based teaching, medical ethics and law, and widening participation issues.

Series Editors

Katharine Boursicot is a reader in Medical Education and Deputy Head of the Centre for Medical and Healthcare Education at St George's, University of London. Previously she was Head of Assessment at Barts and The London, and Associate Dean for Assessment for Cambridge University School of Medicine. She is consultant on assessment to several UK medical schools, Royal Colleges, and international institutions, as well as the General Medical Council Professional and Linguistic Assessment Boards Part 2 panel and fitness to practise clinical skills testing.

David Sales is a General Practitioner by training who has been involved in medical assessment for over 20 years, having previously been convenor of the MRCGP knowledge test. He has run item writing workshops for a number of undergraduate medical schools, medical Royal Colleges, and internationally. For the General Medical Council he currently chairs the Professional and Linguistic Assessment Boards Part 1 panel and is their consultant on fitness to practise knowledge testing.

Contributors

Joy Bell
Specialty Trainee in General Adult Psychiatry, Northern Ireland

Mark Broadhurst
Consultant Psychiatrist, Derbyshire Healthcare NHS Foundation Trust

Esra Caglar
Child and Adolescent Psychiatrist and Specialty Trainee in Medical Psychotherapy, Tavistock and Portman NHS Foundation Trust

Kelly Clarke
MB PhD student with a special interest in global mental health, UCL Institute for Global Health

Tim Exworthy
Consultant Forensic Psychiatrist and Clinical Director Men's Service, St Andrew's Healthcare, Northampton

Susannah Fairweather
Consultant Child and Adolescent Psychiatrist, Tavistock and Portman NHS Foundation Trust

Amber Fossey
Specialty Trainee in Forensic Psychiatry, West London Mental Health Trust

Holly Greer
Specialty Trainee in Learning Disability Psychiatry, Belfast Trust, Northern Ireland

Jonathan Hill
Professor of Child and Adolescent Psychiatry, University of Manchester,Honorary Consultant Psychiatrist, Central Manchester NHS Foundation Trust, and Tavistock and Portman NHS Foundation Trust

Andrew Horton
Consultant Psychiatrist, Derbyshire Healthcare NHS Foundation Trust

Kazuya Iwata
Honorary Clinical Lecturer, Academic Centre for Medical Education, UCLMS, and Consultant Psychiatrist, Southeast Newham Sector

Greg Lydall
Consultant Psychiatrist in Adult Psychiatry with a special interest in Substance Misuse, Castel Hospital, Guernsey

Maggie McGurgan
Specialty Trainee in Learning Disability Psychiatry, Belfast Trust, Northern Ireland

Louise Morganstein
Specialty Trainee in Child and Adolescent Psychiatry, Tavistock and Portman NHS Foundation Trust

Paula Murphy
Consultant Forensic Psychiatrist, St Andrew's Healthcare, Northampton

Peter Sloan
Locum Consultant in Unscheduled Care Team, Belfast Health and Social Care Trust

Julian Summerfield
Consultant in General Adult Psychiatry, Camden and Islington NHS Foundation Trust

Clare Wadlow
Clinical Teaching Fellow and
Specialty Registrar in Old Age
Psychiatry, Academic Centre for
Medical Education, University
College London.

Andrew Watson
Consultant Psychiatrist and
Honorary Senior Lecturer,
Edinburgh University

Michael Yousif
Consultant in Psychological
Medicine, Oxford University
Hospitals NHS Trust

Abbreviations

ABG	arterial blood gas
ACT	acceptance and commitment therapy
ADH	antidiuretic hormone
ADHD	attention deficit hyperactivity disorder
ADL	activities of daily living
AIDS	acquired immunodeficiency syndrome
ASD	autism spectrum disorders
bd	bis die (Latin)—twice daily
BDD	body dysmorphic disorder
BMI	body mass index
BP	blood pressure
BPAD	bipolar affective disorder
bpm	beats per minute
CAMHS	Child and Adolescent Mental Health Services
CAT	cognitive analytic therapy
CBT	cognitive behavioural therapy
CGAS	Children's Global Assessment Scale
CK	creatine kinase
CMHT	community mental health team
CNS	central nervous system
COMT	catechol-O-methyltransferase
CPN	community psychiatric nurse
CRP	C-reactive protein
CT	computed tomography
DALY	disability-adjusted life years
DBT	dialectic behavioural therapy
DSH	deliberate self-harm
DSM-IV	Diagnostic and Statistical Manual of Mental Disorders, Fourth Edition
DSM-5	Diagnostic and Statistical Manual of Mental Disorders, Fifth Edition
DVLA	Driver and Vehicle Licensing Agency
ECG	electrocardiogram
ECT	electroconvulsive therapy

ED	Emergency Department
EEG	electroencephalogram
EPSE	extrapyramidal side-effect
FAST	Fast Alcohol Screening Test
FBC	full blood count
FRS	first rank symptom
FTD	frontotemporal dementia
FY1	foundation year 1 doctor
GABA	gamma-aminobutyric acid
GCS	Glasgow Coma Scale
GHB	gamma-hydroxybutyrate
GI	gastrointestinal
GMC	General Medical Council
GP	general practitioner
HIV	human immunodeficiency virus
HoNOSCA	Health of the Nation Outcome Scales for Children and Adolescents
ICD-10	International Statistical Classification of Diseases and Related Health Problems 10th Revision
IM	intramuscular
IPT	interpersonal therapy
IQ	intelligence quotient
ITU	intensive treatment unit
IV	intravenous
LD	learning difficulty
LFT	liver function test
LSD	lysergic acid diethylamide
LTM	long-term memory
mane	in the morning
MAOI	monoamine oxidase inhibitor
MDMA	3,4-methylenedioxy-N-methylamphetamine
MDT	multidisciplinary team
MFQ	Mood and Feelings Questionnaire
MHA	Mental Health Act
MMSE®-2™	Mini-Mental State Examination
MRI	magnetic resonance imaging
MSE	Mental State Examination
MSU	mid-stream urine
MUS	medically unexplained symptoms

NHS	National Health Service
NICE	National Institute for Health and Clinical Excellence
NMDA	N-methyl-D-aspartate
NMS	neuroleptic malignant syndrome
nocte	at nighttime
NR	nearest relative
OCD	obsessive-compulsive disorder
od	omni die (Latin)—daily
OHCM	*Oxford Handbook of Clinical Medicine*
OHPsych	*Oxford Handbook of Psychiatry*
OT	occupational therapist
PCP	phencyclidine
PD	personality disorder
PKU	phenylketonuria
PO	per os (Latin)—by mouth, orally
PRN	pro re nata (Latin)—as required
PTSD	post-traumatic stress disorder
qds	quarter die sumendus (Latin)—four times a day
RC	Responsible Clinician
RCPsych	Royal College of Psychiatrists
RCT	randomized controlled trial
REM	rapid eye movement
rINN	recommended International Non-Proprietary Name
RIOTT	Randomised Injectable Opiate Treatment Trial
RTC	road traffic collision
SALT	speech and language therapist
SDQ	Strengths and Difficulties Questionnaire
SNRI	serotonin–noradrenaline reuptake inhibitor
SSRI	selective serotonin reuptake inhibitor
STM	short-term memory
TCA	tricyclic antidepressants
tds	ter die sumendus (Latin)—three times a day
TFTs	thyroid function tests
TLE	temporal lobe epilepsy
TS	tuberous sclerosis
TSH	thyroid stimulating hormone
U&Es	urea and electrolytes
UCLMS	University College London Medical School
UDS	urinary drug screen

URTI	upper respiratory tract infection
UTI	urinary tract infection
VCFS	velo-cardio-facial syndrome
WHO	World Health Organization
WCC	white cell count
YBOCS	Yale–Brown Obsessive Compulsive Scale

How To Use This Book

Oxford Assess and Progress: Psychiatry has been carefully designed to ensure you get the most out of your revision and are prepared for your exams. Here is a brief guide to some of the features and learning tools.

Organization of content

Chapter editorials will help you unpick tricky subjects, and when it's late at night and you need something to remind you why you're doing this, you'll find words of encouragement!

Chapters begin with Single Best Answer (SBAs) questions followed by Extended Matching Questions (EMQs). Answers can be found at the end of each chapter, beginning with the SBA answers and then the EMQ answers.

How to read an answer

Unlike other revision guides on the market, this one is crammed full of feedback, so you should understand exactly why each answer is correct, and gain an insight into the common pitfalls. With every answer there is an explanation of why that particular choice is the most appropriate. For some questions there is additional explanation of why the distracters are less suitable. Where relevant you will also be directed to sources of further information, such as the *Oxford Handbook of Clinical Specialties*, websites, and journal articles.

→ http://www.bmj.com/cgi/content/full/334/7583/35?grp = 1

Progression points

The questions in every chapter are ordered by level of difficulty and competence, indicated by the following symbols:

★   Graduate 'should know'—you should be aiming to get most of these correct.
★★   Graduate 'nice to know'—these are a bit tougher but not above your capabilities.
★★★   Foundation Doctor 'should know'—these will really test your understanding.
★★★★   Foundation Doctor 'nice to know'—give these a go when you're ready to challenge yourself.

Oxford Handbook of Psychiatry

The *Oxford Handbook of Psychiatry* (OHPsych) page references are given with the answers to some questions, e.g. OHPsych 3rd edn → p.340. Please note that this reference is to the **3rd Edition** of the OHPsych, and that subsequent editions are unlikely to have the same material in exactly the same place.

Chapter 1

Descriptive psychopathology

Julian Summerfield and Michael Yousif

Psychopathology is 'the systematic study of abnormal experience, cognition and behaviour; the study of the products of a disordered mind' (Sims, 2002). *Descriptive psychopathology* refers to a particular approach to the assessment and understanding of the signs and symptoms of mental disorder and forms the basis of clinical psychiatry. The term *descriptive* in this context refers to a necessarily value- and theory-free interpretation of the mental and behavioural phenomena a patient presents with. For students of medicine and psychiatry, it is essential to understand the significance of this and the rationale behind it.

Psychiatry is unique among the medical specialties in that there are few objective clinical signs and no biomarkers (at least *in vivo*) which indicate the presence or otherwise of specific mental disorders. Contrast this with bodily disorders whose features are physical and objective; they lend themselves to being measurable, quantifiable, and therefore reliable to assess. Features of mental disorders present through behaviour and experience (thoughts, feelings, perceptions); they are internal and essentially subjective. This renders psychopathological phenomena elusive to clinical assessment in the way physical disorders are, leaving psychiatry in somewhat of a quandary; how to establish a reliable and valid system of assessing subjective phenomena? Furthermore, there needs to be a safeguard against the undue influence of bias caused by personal value judgements when interpreting subjective phenomenon. A chest X-ray showing a lobe consolidation or a blood test showing anaemia is open to far less interpretation than a person complaining of low mood or hearing voices.

A further challenge in addition to that posed by the subjective nature of psychopathological phenomena is that of the absence of established aetiological mechanisms of mental disorders. Whether they are caused by physical changes in the brain or are social phenomena caused by experience (or some combination) remains contentious. Indeed, this debate continues to strike at the very concept of mental disorder.

Therefore, clinical assessment of a person presenting with mental disorder must enable accessing and understanding the patient's inner world; it must be based on a system that is value-free so as to avoid the undue influence of the personal beliefs of the clinician; and it obviously cannot be reliant on thus-far absent aetiology. In order to meet these requirements, psychiatric assessment becomes based on a neutral *description* of a patient's experiences and behaviour. These features are elicited through specialist observation and communication skills.

A descriptive approach can be contrasted with an *explanatory* approach, which is based on aetiology. Explanatory systems of pathology can and do exist in physical medicine. A given sign or symptom of mental disorder may well be associated with a diagnosis, such as delusions with schizophrenia, low mood with depression, or palpitations with anxiety; but this association does not imply an *aetiological* mechanism. Descriptive psychopathology therefore informs clinicians of the various manifestations of mental disorders. It constitutes the system of eliciting the present signs and symptoms of mental disorder through the *Mental State Examination* (MSE), which remains the core clinical skill of the psychiatrist.

Julian Summerfield and Michael Yousif

QUESTIONS

Single Best Answers

1. A 29-year-old woman with bipolar affective disorder (BPAD) has been closely monitored in the community by her mental health team due to a hypomanic relapse. Concerns are raised at the team meeting that this may be developing into a manic episode. Which is the *single* most indicative symptom of this new change? ★

A Elevation of mood

B Flight of ideas

C Increased energy levels

D Overfamiliarity

E Reduced sleep

2. A 71-year-old man has become increasingly distressed over the last 24 hours. He is agitated and thought-disordered with tangential thinking. He states that his son, who lives in France, has been trying to poison him. He says that he can see his son standing at the end of his bed laughing at him. He becomes angry when told that his son is not there. Which is the *single* most diagnostic symptom for organic pathology? ★

A Agitation

B Paranoid delusions

C Poor insight

D Thought disorder

E Visual hallucinations

3. A 45-year-old man, who is one day post-elective cholecystectomy, is aggressive and is demanding to leave the ward. He had brief contact with local alcohol services three years ago. He is agitated, tremulous, fearful, confused, and paranoid. Which is the *single* most likely perceptual abnormality that he will have? ★

A Gustatory hallucinations

B Olfactory hallucinations

C Tactile hallucinations

D Third-person auditory hallucinations

E Visual hallucinations

4. A 28-year-old woman repeatedly brings her one-month-old baby to the Emergency Department (ED). On each occasion she states that she is worried that she has accidentally harmed her baby by giving him the wrong formula. She says that she knows these thoughts are 'silly' and she can be reassured, but the worries soon return. She cannot stop thinking about this and is constantly checking her baby for signs of illness. Which is the *single* most appropriate term for her thoughts? ★

A Hypochondriacal delusion

B Illness phobia

C Negative cognition

D Obsession

E Overvalued idea

5. A 23-year-old woman hears muffled voices and poorly defined noises as she is falling asleep. She finds this distressing but denies any other problems. Which is the *single* most appropriate description for this symptom? ★

A Auditory hallucination

B Functional hallucination

C Hypnagogic hallucination

D Hypnopompic hallucination

E Pseudohallucination

6. An unemployed 64-year-old man with alcohol dependence moves to a new area. His daughter reports that he has been experiencing problems with his memory, particularly since moving home. He claims to know the area very well as he says he has lived there for many years and works nearby. However, the descriptions he gives of where he lives and what he does are vague. Which is the *single* most appropriate explanation for his account? ★

A Confabulation

B Confusion

C Delusion

D Fantasy

E Palimpsest

7. A 63-year-old man with paranoid schizophrenia has suffered recurrent episodes of acute psychosis requiring compulsory treatment under the Mental Health Act (MHA). He takes haloperidol and has not had any admissions for seven years. He has recently been exhibiting negative symptoms of schizophrenia. Which is the *single* most likely description of his affect on MSE? ★

A Blunted

B Flattened

C Incongruous

D Labile

E Reactive

8. A 27-year-old woman from the Republic of Congo is seen in outpatients. She reports witnessing and being subjected to multiple abuses before seeking asylum in the UK. She is concerned she may have post-traumatic stress disorder (PTSD). Which is the *single* most suggestive feature of this diagnosis? ★

A Flattened affect

B Increased startle response

C Poor concentration

D Tearfulness

E Unwillingness to discuss her abuses in detail

9. A 23-year-old man has become progressively socially withdrawn and has been neglecting himself over the last six months. He is suspicious that he is being followed by secret service agents. He believes that the government is putting distressing thoughts into his mind as part of an experiment. Recently he has been hearing a voice telling him to kill himself. Which *single* symptom is most indicative of schizophrenia? ★★

A Persecutory delusion

B Second-person auditory hallucinations

C Self-neglect

D Social withdrawal

E Thought insertion

10. A 16-year-old adolescent has lost 10 kg in weight over the past year by restricting her calorie intake and exercising excessively. Her body mass index (BMI) is now 16 kg/m². She has been feeling faint at school and has not had a period for four months. She believes that she is much bigger than her classmates and is constantly afraid that she will put on weight. Which is the *single* most appropriate description for this belief? ★★

A Delusion

B Dysmorphophobia

C Obsession

D Overvalued idea

E Preoccupation

11. A 25-year-old man with schizophrenia on an acute psychiatric ward lacks motivation, walks very slowly, says very little, and often stands still for long periods. When his arms are moved into a posture, he holds them there until they are moved again. He is thought to have developed catatonia. Which *single* clinical finding is most supportive of this diagnosis? ★★

A Alogia

B Apathy

C Bradykinesia

D Cogwheel rigidity

E Waxy flexibility

12. A 27-year-old man has consumed large quantities of cocaine and is now acutely agitated and hostile in the ED. Which is the *single* most likely perceptual abnormality he will have? ★★

A Auditory hallucination

B Gustatory hallucination

C Olfactory hallucination

D Tactile hallucination

E Visual hallucination

13. A 28-year-old woman falls and abruptly starts shaking her legs and arms for 30 seconds. She appears acutely distressed during the episode. Since the death of her mother three months ago, she has experienced several of these episodes during the day. Which *single* finding supports a diagnosis of pseudoseizure as opposed to epilepsy? ★★

A Absence of rigidity prior to limb jerking

B Absence of urinating during the seizure

C Expression of distress

D Rapid onset and termination

E Short time length

14. A 35-year-old woman has features associated with atypical depression. Which is the *single* most likely finding on MSE? ★★

A Flattened affect

B Insomnia

C Negative thoughts about the future

D Psychomotor agitation

E Weight gain

15. A 21-year-old woman has had recurrent 'strange episodes' lasting approximately five minutes over the last six months. She is given a provisional diagnosis of temporal lobe epilepsy (TLE). Which *single* symptom is most indicative of this diagnosis? ★★★

A Auditory hallucinations

B Automatisms

C Depersonalization

D Euphoria

E Formal thought disorder

16. A 19-year-old man says that he is sometimes able to taste the music and hear the colours when watching pop music videos. Which is the *single* most appropriate description of this experience? ★★★

A Auditory hallucination

B Delusional perception

C Gustatory hallucination

D Illusion

E Synaesthesia

17. A 77-year-old woman, who has been living alone since the death of her husband seven years ago, has developed severe memory loss over the last six months. She feels that her short- and long-term memories (STM and LTM) are severely affected. She also has poor sleep and has lost at least 10 kg in the last year. Her Mini-Mental State Examination (MMSE®-2™) score is 18/23: she is fully orientated but unable to complete the exam and loses points mainly because of her markedly reduced concentration span. Which is the *single* most support-ive feature of a pseudodementia in this patient? ★★★

A Bereavement

B MMSE®-2™ performance

C Poor sleep

D STM and LTM affected

E Weight loss

18. A 69-year-old woman with longstanding recurrent depressive disorder has had low mood, anhedonia, lethargy, and insomnia for the past two months. More recently she has begun to believe that her bowels are rotting inside her. Which is the *single* most appropriate description of this mood-congruent delusion? ★★★★

A Capgras syndrome

B Cotard syndrome

C Couvade syndrome

D Frégoli syndrome

E Othello syndrome

19. A 65-year-old man with chronic schizophrenia is suspected of suffering acute frontal lobe injury. Which *single* finding is most supportive of this diagnosis? ★★★★

A Apathy

B Concrete thinking

C Disinhibition

D Inattention

E Perseveration

20. A 67-year-old man has had progressive cognitive impairment over the last year. His brother was diagnosed with cortical dementia four years ago and he is convinced he has this as well. The memory team suspect he has subcortical dementia instead. Which *single* clinical feature is most indicative of this alternative diagnosis? ★★★★

A Amnesia

B Aphasia

C Apraxia

D Depression

E Inattention

Extended Matching Questions

Delusions

For each scenario below, choose the *single* most appropriate type of delusion from the list of options. Each option may be used once, more than once, or not at all. ★

A Delusional mood

B Delusion of control

C Delusion of misidentification

D Delusion of thought insertion

E Grandiose delusion

F Hypochondriacal delusion

G Nihilistic delusion

H Paranoid delusion

I Partition delusion

J Persecutory delusion

1. A 32-year-old man feels a general yet definite sense that his sur-
roundings have changed in a way that is profoundly relevant for
him, and that something significant is impending.

2. A 71-year-old woman believes people are entering her house
through the walls in order to poison her food.

3. A 33-year-old man believes his intestines have rotted away and no
longer exist.

4. A 27-year-old woman believes all news articles are referring to her
in some hidden but definite way.

5. A 66-year-old man believes a secret organization is tampering with
his food and making him seriously ill.

Frontotemporal dementia (FTD) speech content

For each scenario below, choose the *single* most appropriate term from the list of options. Each option may be used once, more than once, or not at all. ★

A Circumstantiality

B Clanging

C Derailment

D Flight of ideas

E Neologisms

F Phonemic paraphasia

G Poverty of content of speech

H Poverty of speech

I Tangentiality

J Word salad

6. A 27-year-old man with schizophrenia is observed to be self-neglecting. When asked about this, and other questions, he responds with long, rambling passages of speech which convey little meaningful information.

7. A 29-year-old woman with BPAD is having a hypomanic episode. She is engaging and cooperative but slightly distractible. She displays a speech pattern that remains on-topic but, perhaps due to her distractibility, is more indirect and incorporates a lot of talking around the subject before eventually reaching the goal.

8. A 24-year-old man with schizophrenia has been smoking significant amounts of cannabis recently. It is difficult to understand what he is saying as his speech jumps from one topic to another with no apparent connection between topics.

9. A 40-year-old man with schizophrenia has recently stopped taking his medication. He engages well in clinical interview, but when replying to some questions he quickly moves off-topic although his answer is tenuously related to the question.

10. A 35-year-old woman is thought to be suffering from a psychotic illness. She does not appear able to answer any questions. Instead her speech pattern seems to be more governed by the sound of the words rather than their meaning.

ANSWERS

Single Best Answers

1. B ★   OHPsych 3rd edn → pp.306–8

The most indicative symptom of mania is (B). The difference between hypomania, a milder version of illness, and mania may be one of degree. However, psychotic symptoms such as thought disorder (including flight of ideas) represent a categorical difference in severity between them and will only occur in mania. Flight of ideas is a type of disorder of the form (i.e. structure) of thought. Thought disorder is a psychotic symptom, which denotes the presence of full-blown mania. With flight of ideas, the patient's direction of thinking fluctuates rapidly. One thought jumps rapidly to the next, with a logical but loose association.

Mood elevation (A) in the context of BPAD may typically manifest in persistent cheerfulness or exuberance that is disproportionate to the context. It can be present in hypomania and mania, depending on the degree.

Increased energy levels (C) could be present in hypomania and mania, depending on the degree. They might also be due to other reasons that are non-psychiatric in nature, such as being in a new relationship, or a new job, or even the season (people tend to feel more energetic when the sun is out, compared to a dark, rainy day).

Overfamiliarity (D) towards others may manifest in increased sociability or overstepping normal interpersonal boundaries. It can be present in hypomania and mania, depending on the degree.

Reduced sleep (E) could be present in hypomania and mania, depending on the degree. This symptom can also be present in depression.

2. E ★   OHPsych 3rd edn → pp.134–5

Visual hallucinations (E) tend to occur in organic states rather than functional psychoses such as schizophrenia, and are therefore most indicative of an organic psychosis. Paranoid delusions, thought disorder, and poor insight are all potential symptoms of a psychotic illness. However, given the sudden onset of the presentation in an elderly man with no reported previous psychiatric history, an organic cause must be considered in the first instance. In this case, you would seek to identify other signs and symptoms suggestive of organic pathology, such as clouding of consciousness, disorientation, and neurological signs. Following a full physical examination, appropriate investigations may include blood tests, urine dipstick, electrocardiogram (ECG), and brain imaging.

Agitation (A) is often exhibited by people suffering with dementias or delirium. However, it is a non-specific sign that may also arise in non-organic functional psychiatric disorders. It is, of course, also a normal behaviour in many situations and not necessarily psychopathological.

Paranoid (which in psychiatry technically means self-referential, not necessarily persecutory) delusions can arise in any psychotic illness, regardless of aetiology. The common use of the term 'paranoid delusion', where someone describes being followed, spied on, or in danger, is actually a delusion subset called persecutory paranoid delusions (B).

Insight (C) is the ability of a person to understand the nature and effect of their own mental health. Poor insight can also arise in any psychotic illness, regardless of aetiology. Insight is part of a continuum, rather than a present/absent dichotomy, and should be assessed as such through careful exploration.

Formal thought disorders (D) are recognized as changes in speech, writing, or occasionally behaviour due to difficulties in thought form. This means the 'form' or way the thoughts are used rather than their content. Formal thought disorder can arise in many different psychotic illnesses, regardless of aetiology. These disorders are also seen in times of extreme stress or intoxication.

→ Horn H, Federspiel A, Wirth M, *et al.* (2009). Structural and metabolic changes in language areas linked to formal thought disorder. *British Journal of Psychiatry*, **194**, 130–8.

3. E ★   OHPsych 3rd edn → p.570

This presentation is suggestive of a delirium tremens, an acute confusional state secondary to alcohol withdrawal. The patient has no reported psychiatric history and there is a suggestion of excessive alcohol use in the past. Since coming in for elective surgery, he would have had no access to alcohol which may have precipitated a withdrawal state. It would be important to gather further history from the patient or other sources regarding his previous and recent alcohol use. Delirium tremens is a medical emergency with a mortality of up to 10% due to the risk of seizures and dehydration. The differential diagnosis here would include intoxication, acute functional psychotic illness, or a delirium with another primary cause such as infection. Visual hallucinations (E) are characteristic of organic states. In particular with delirium tremens, the patient may experience visual 'Lilliputian' hallucinations of small people (after the Lilliputs in *Gulliver's Travels* by Jonathan Swift) or small animals (one classic example is seeing pink elephants).

Gustatory (taste) hallucinations (A) may occur in schizophrenia and also in some organic states such as TLE.

Olfactory (smell) hallucinations (B) may occur in schizophrenia and also in some organic states such as Parkinson's disease.

Tactile hallucinations (C) may arise in a range of organic states, including delirium tremens and cocaine intoxication (so-called 'formication' is the sensation of insects crawling on the skin).

Third-person auditory hallucinations (D) are a first rank symptom (FRS) of schizophrenia, and therefore more indicative of functional illness.

→ http://en.wikipedia.org/wiki/lilliput_and_blefuscu

4. D ★   OHPsych 3rd edn → pp.376–8

The answer is an obsession (D). This is an unpleasant, intrusive, and repetitive thought that is recognized as irrational and as the patient's own. The thought often leads to increasing anxiety which is relieved by a compulsion or safety behaviour (in this example, the mother engages in compulsive checking for signs of illness and taking the child to the ED). However, reassurance from the compulsions only provides temporary relief from anxiety.

A delusion (A) is a fixed, false belief that is held with absolute conviction and despite any evidence to the contrary, and that is not in keeping with a person's cultural background and beliefs. Therefore, a hypochondriacal delusion involves the belief that one has already acquired a particular disease despite evidence to the contrary. In the case given above, the patient is able to recognize that her belief is irrational and can be reassured, albeit temporarily.

A phobia (B) is an excessive fear of a particular object or situation that leads to profound anticipatory anxiety and avoidance. An illness phobia would therefore involve an unreasonable fear about developing an illness associated with measures to avoid situations that are perceived as risky (for example, avoiding public transport in case of exposure to a communicable disease).

Negative cognitions (C) are negative thoughts that occur in depression. Aaron Beck proposed a triad of negative thoughts in depression concerning the self, the world, and the future. So, a person with depression may believe they are worthless, that others dislike them because they are worthless, and they are hopeless that their situation will change.

An overvalued idea (E) is a false belief that causes excessive preoccupation and distress. In terms of the degree of conviction with which it is held, it can be considered on the spectrum of delusions but is less fixed, and this is what differentiates it from a psychotic delusion.

5. C ★   OHPsych 3rd edn → pp.56–7

The answer is an hallucination that occurs while falling asleep, known as a hypnagogic hallucination (C). The experience may be auditory, visual, or tactile and the person may be woken by the hallucination. This is often confused with a hypnopompic hallucination, so memorize it by remembering hypna*GO*gic hallucinations occur when you are *GO*ing to sleep.

An hallucination is a sensory perceptual experience without an external stimulus. It can arise in any sensory modality. It is a psychotic symptom and can be caused by both functional and organic psychiatric disorders. It is perceived as real by the person and subjective reality testing does not distinguish the experience from a true perceptual experience. An auditory hallucination is the false perception of a sound without a corresponding external stimulus (A).

A functional hallucination (B) is a false perception experienced alongside a normal stimulus in the same sensory modality; for example, a patient hearing voices whenever they hear the wind blowing through a tree.

An hallucination that occurs when waking up is known as a hypnopompic hallucination (D). Both hypnagogic and hypnopompic hallucinations can occur in healthy people and are not necessarily a sign of mental illness. They have also been described in narcolepsy, delirium, depression, anxiety, and drug intoxication such as glue sniffing.

A pseudohallucination (E) is a false perception that is experienced in subjective internal space and is not concretely regarded as real. For example, a depressed person describes hearing a negative voice inside their head which, on further exploration, they recognize as their own. Pseudohallucinations can occur in any sensory modality and have an 'as if' quality. They may occur in psychotic, organic, or drug-induced states, in personality disorder (PD), or they can be a normal experience in times of crisis or bereavement.

6. A ★   OHPsych 3rd edn → pp.89, 566

The answer is confabulation (A). This man is possibly suffering from Korsakoff's psychosis which is characterized by anterograde amnesia (an inability to lay down new memories) as well as some retrograde amnesia. It is caused by thiamine deficiency secondary to chronic alcohol abuse and is often preceded by an acute episode of Wernicke's encephalopathy with its classic tetrad of acute confusion, ataxia, nystagmus, and ophthalmoplegia. However, the differential diagnosis in this situation would include acute intoxication, an acute confusional state, or another cause of dementia. Confabulation is the expression of plausible false memories covering up periods of amnesia. The descriptions are often vague and the patient may not be consciously aware that they are imagining these details. Confabulation is a prominent feature of Korsakoff's psychosis but can occur in other forms of dementia.

In an acute confusional state (B) or delirium a patient will usually be disorientated, with clouding of consciousness. Confusion can cause someone to lose the ability to understand what is happening around them, to think rationally, or to store new memories.

A delusion (C) is a fixed, false belief that is held with absolute conviction despite evidence to the contrary, and that would not be shared by other people from the same culture, religion, or community. This does not describe what this man is exhibiting.

A fantasy (D) is an imagined situation in which an individual expresses certain desires or aims. Fantasy is a term commonly used in psychoanalysis: Sigmund Freud saw the fantasy as an imaginary wish fulfilment.

Palimpsest (E) is the term for amnesia related to a discrete period of alcohol or drug intoxication. It is sometimes referred to as a 'blackout', although while intoxicated the person had not lost consciousness and appeared to be functioning normally. Palimpsest is more common while intoxicated in the context of chronic alcohol abuse.

7. A ★   OHPysch 3rd edn → pp.178–9

The answer is a blunted affect (A), which is where there is a narrowed affective response, where the person shows little mood reactivity to any given stimulus. This is characteristic of chronic schizophrenia. It should be noted, however, that on observation it can be difficult to distinguish from the parkinsonian side-effects of long-term neuroleptic use (such as bradykinesia or expressionless face).

A flattened affect (B) is congruous with a depressed mood. The person will persistently exhibit this even when confronted with positive stimuli. It is important to note that it can be difficult to distinguish between a flattened and blunted affect, but it is important to be aware of the distinctive phenomenology.

An incongruous affect (C) is where, for example, a person may be laughing while describing something traumatic—or vice versa. This is more typical of acute psychosis.

A labile affect (D) is where a person's affective response is congruous and appropriate to the given stimulus, but which switches rapidly in a short space of time and may be disproportionate to the prevailing context.

A reactive affect (E) is one where there is a proportionate and appropriate response to the given contact or stimulus. It may indicate euthymia, but can also be present in milder forms of psychosis or mood disorder.

→ Liddle PF (2007). Schizophrenia: the clinical picture. In G Stein and G Wilkinson (eds), *Seminars in General Adult Psychiatry*, pp. 167–8. Royal College of Psychiatrists, London.

8. B ★   OHPsych 3rd edn → pp.390–1

Features of hyperarousal constitute a diagnostic criterion of PTSD. Hyperarousal can manifest in an increased startle response (B), insomnia, irritability, and poor concentration.

A flattened affect (A) is more indicative of depression. In PTSD, people may experience a reduced capacity to exhibit emotions, which may present as a restricted affect.

Poor concentration (C) is a non-specific sign and could indicate a range of mental health problems, including depression and anxiety.

Tearfulness (D) is also a non-specific sign, and could be part of a normal emotional reaction.

PTSD can cause partial amnesia around the traumatic event. This must be distinguished from a volitional unwillingness to discuss details (E), which may be wholly understandable in the context.

9. E ★★   OHPsych 3rd edn → pp.178–9

Thought insertion (E) is an FRS. Though not pathognomic (it can be present in manic psychoses, for example), its presence is highly suggestive of schizophrenia.

The German psychiatrist, Kurt Schneider, described a number of 'symptoms of first rank' in the acute phase of schizophrenia. FRSs constitute core features of the illness and are most indicative of the disorder:

- Third-person auditory hallucinations, thought echo, running commentary
- Thought insertion, withdrawal, broadcast
- Passivity—somatic, affect, impulse, volition
- Delusional perception

Persecutory delusions (A), such as the belief that one is being followed by government agents, are common in schizophrenia but are not an FRS.

Second-person auditory hallucinations (B) where the voice is talking to the person, though common in schizophrenia, are not FRSs. Third-person auditory hallucinations where the voice is talking about the person, are FRS.

Self-neglect (C) is a common feature of many mental disorders. It is common in schizophrenia and may be a negative symptom of the illness.

There are many reasons why this man may have withdrawn from his social groups, most of which are not related to a mental illness. For example, if he were starting to question his sexuality while in a community that does not accept homosexuality, this may lead to an abrupt withdrawal and move to a different social group. It may, however, be part of something more worrying, and therefore careful assessment is needed.

→ Mellor CS (1970). First rank symptoms of schizophrenia. *British Journal of Psychiatry*, **117**, 15–23.

10. D ★★   OHPsych 3rd edn → pp.101, 398–9

The answer is overvalued ideas (D); these are abnormal beliefs that are acceptable and understandable but are pursued unreasonably by the patient and come to dominate their life. An overvalued idea is held with less intensity or conviction than a delusion. A core feature of anorexia is the overvalued idea in the form of body image distortion (that one is overweight) or morbid fear of fatness, which is intrusive and leads to significant distress or functional impairment.

A diagnosis of anorexia nervosa can be made on the basis of low weight (BMI < 17.5 kg/m²), self-induced weight loss (for example, by calorie restriction, avoidance of fattening foods, overexercise, or use of appetite suppressants, diuretics, or laxatives), and endocrine dysfunction (in this case amenorrhoea). The usual psychopathology includes overvalued ideas such as a dread of fatness and body image distortion (the patient believes they are fat when they are actually underweight). A delusion (A) is a fixed, false belief that is held with absolute conviction despite evidence to the contrary and is not shared by other members of the same community or culture. It can be hard to distinguish between a delusion and an overvalued idea. Delusions are more likely to have an abrupt onset and implausible content, and the deluded individual may be relatively indifferent to the opinions of others.

Dysmorphophobia (B) is a fixation on an imaginary flaw in physical appearance and is often is encountered in dermatology and cosmetic surgery settings. Dysmorphophobic symptoms in a dermatology setting have been termed dermatological hypochondriasis. As with hypochondriasis, it is a persistent, false belief or worry. The key features are the preoccupation with the deformity, along with repeatedly seeking reassurance despite evidence, such as repeated tests. Even in cases where a minor defect truly exists, there is an inordinate amount of anguish and fixation on the flaw.

An obsession (C) is a repetitive, unpleasant, intrusive thought that is recognized as the patient's own. It is experienced subjectively as senseless, which distinguishes it from a delusion or overvalued idea.

A preoccupation (E) is a thought that dominates the mind to the exclusion of all else. It may not be an abnormal belief and therefore does not necessarily denote psychopathology.

11. E ★★   OHPsych 3rd edn → p.88

The answer is waxy flexibility (E), a form of posturing seen in catatonia. When the patient's arms are moved into a posture by the examiner, they will be retained in that position for several minutes at least. Two other forms of unusual posturing seen in catatonia are stereotypy (where bizarre and uncomfortable postures are adopted for hours) and psychological pillow (where the patient keeps his head slightly raised when lying down, as if resting on a non-existent pillow).

Catatonia has been less prevalent since the advent of antipsychotic medication and earlier intervention in psychosis. Characteristic signs include posturing, mutism, staring, negativism (resisting all instructions of movements), echopraxia (the patient imitates the interviewer's actions), and rigidity (which is abolished by active or passive movement). Alogia (A), or poverty of speech, is a negative symptom of schizophrenia. It occurs in the absence of catatonia. The lack of spontaneous speech hints at an underlying poverty of thoughts.

Apathy (B) is another negative symptom of schizophrenia, along with avolition, blunted affect, and lack of drive. It is important to remember that patients may be over-sedated because of their medication or suffering with co-morbid depression, which can present as apathy.

Bradykinesia (C), which means moving slowly, is a parkinsonian symptom. It can be an extrapyramidal side-effect (EPSE) of antipsychotic medication, along with tremor and rigidity. Other EPSEs are acute dystonia, akathisia, and tardive dyskinesia.

Cogwheel rigidity (D) is the combination of tremor and rigidity felt when an examiner moves a patient's limb. Tremor and rigidity may both be due to EPSEs, and cogwheel rigidity is distinct from the rigidity seen in catatonia which disappears on active or passive movement.

→ World Health Organization (1992). *The ICD-10 Classification of Mental and Behavioural Disorders*. WHO, Geneva. http://www.who.int/classifications/icd/en/.

12. D ★★   OHPsych 3rd edn → pp.56–7

The answer is tactile hallucinations (D), such as 'formication', the hallucination of feeling insects crawling on one's skin, which is classically associated with cocaine intoxication.

Cocaine is a sympathomimetic drug, through enhancing the effects of monoamine neurotransmitters such as dopamine and noradrenaline in the synaptic clefts. Chronic use or acute intoxication can lead to the development of a range of psychotic symptoms. Cocaine can lead to auditory hallucinations (A), though these may be more classically associated with amphetamine-based drugs which can produce schizophreniform psychoses.

Gustatory hallucinations (B) would be unusual in recreational drug intoxication. They are usually present in organic disorders such as TLE and in schizophrenia.

Olfactory hallucinations (C) would also be unusual in recreational drug intoxication. They are usually present in organic disorders such as Parkinson's disease. If there is a distortion in olfaction then assessment should be made to differentiate between distortions due to inhaled odorants (troposmia) and distortions when there are no odorants in the environment (phantosmia).

Visual hallucinations (E) are less common in cocaine intoxication. These would be more in keeping with lysergic acid diethylamide (LSD) which is known to cause 'trips' and it is this effect that is sought by some drug users. These are also seen with phencyclidine and ecstasy.

13. C ★★   OHPsych 3rd edn → pp.806–7

The answer is expression of distress (C). Tonic-clonic seizures are generalized seizures. In generalized seizures there is loss of consciousness. An expression of distress during the episode indicates some degree of conscious awareness. It is notoriously difficult to distinguish between pseudoseizures and epileptic seizures solely on the basis of observation as there are no features specific to either aetiology. A further complicating factor is that, as some studies estimate, as many as 40% of people with epilepsy also experience pseudoseizures. Further investigations with electroencephalogram (EEG) and video telemetry are usually required to help make the distinction.

Tonic-clonic seizures are usually characterized by a brief period of tonic rigidity followed by the limb shaking. The absence of this feature, however, does not rule out epilepsy (A).

Similarly, though urinating and other phenomena such as tongue biting are classically associated with tonic-clonic seizures, this is not consistent and their absence does not preclude a diagnosis of epilepsy (B).

Rapid onset and termination is not the correct answer (D); the timing of the episode alone is not enough on its own to differentiate epilepsy from other types of seizure.

Short time length is also incorrect (E); generalized seizures are commonly associated with some sort of warning and distinctive post-ictal phenomena, but this is not a consistent finding in epilepsy.

→ OHCM 8th edn → p.496

14. E ★★   OHPsych 3rd edn → p.262

Increased appetite and weight gain (E) are often found in atypical depression. Atypical depression is around three times more common in women than in men.

Atypical depression is, as the name suggests, a form of depressive illness which does not present with the classic features of depression such as insomnia, loss of appetite, and weight loss, and affective flattening (A). Atypical depression is characterized by mood/affective reactivity and increased sensitivity to social rejection.

Hypersomnia is more indicative of atypical depression than insomnia (B) or early-morning waking.

Atypical depression is usually characterized by increased sensitivity to social rejection rather than the classic triad which involves negative thoughts about the self (worthlessness), the world (helplessness), and the future (hopelessness) (C).

Feeling weighed down, or classically 'leaden paralysis', is more usual in atypical depression rather than psychomotor agitation (D). Psychomotor agitation can be described as anxiety-related activity such as pacing the room or wringing the hands.

15. B ★★★   OHPsych 3rd edn → pp.156–8

The answer is automatisms (B), which are common in TLE. They are stereotyped movements which are often disorganized and purposeless. The patient is unaware of what they are doing and does not remember their actions afterwards.

There can be a number of psychiatric symptoms linked to epilepsy. TLE results in complex partial seizures and can present with an aura, derealization or depersonalization experiences, cognitive symptoms such as déjà or jamais vu, affective (mood) symptoms, and automatisms or aggressive behaviour during the seizure. TLE also can present with auditory (A), visual, sensory, or olfactory hallucinations, but these can also occur in a number of other psychiatric and organic conditions.

Depersonalization (C) can occur in TLE, other psychiatric disorders, and in healthy people. The patient experiences the sensation that they are not real. In derealization the patient feels that the world around them has become unreal.

Patients with TLE may experience symptoms of anxiety or euphoria (D) in the pre-ictal phase. There is an increased risk of depression, mania, and suicide. However, euphoria may occur in other states such as functional mania, drug intoxication, or in healthy people.

Formal thought disorder (E) involves disruption in the form of thought which can occur in schizophrenia. Examples include thought block, derailment, knight's move thinking, loosening of association, and word salad (perhaps the most extreme form of thought disorder where words are jumbled together in a meaningless way).

→ OHCM 8th edn → pp.494–7

16. E ★★★   OHPsych 3rd edn → p.104

The answer is synaesthesia (E), the experience of a stimulus in one sensory modality being perceived in another sensory modality; for example, hearing a sound that provokes a taste sensation. Synaesthesia may be caused by intoxication with hallucinogenic drugs such as LSD or in epileptic states. However, it is possible for synaesthesia to occur in healthy, normal people, for example in adolescence or at times of crisis or emotional upheaval.

An auditory hallucination (A) is the false perception of a sound without a corresponding external stimulus.

Delusional perception (B) is an FRS of schizophrenia where the patient imbues a normal perception with a delusional meaning. For example, the patient sees the traffic lights change from green to red and, at that precise moment, realizes that this means the world is coming to an end.

Gustatory hallucinations (C) are the perception of a taste without a corresponding external stimulus and they can occur in a variety of conditions such as schizophrenia or TLE, and as a side-effect of psychotropic drugs such as lithium or disulfiram.

An illusion (D) is a false perception that results from the combination of a real-world object and internal imagery, for example, seeing faces in a cloud, mistaking a shadow in a bedroom at night for an intruder, or filling in the gaps to misread an indistinct sign.

→ Hubbard EM (2007). Neurophysiology of synesthesia. *Current Psychiatry Reports*, **9** (3), 193–9.

→ http://web.mit.edu/synesthesia/www/synesthesia.html.

17. B ★★★   OHPsych 3rd edn → pp.102, 520

Being fully orientated in the MMSE®-2™ (B) points away from true cognitive impairment (note the patient lives alone and may have come to the appointment alone, which would indicate a reasonable degree of intact cognition—contrary to her subjective reports).

Bereavement (A) is an incorrect answer. In pseudodementia the cognitive impairment is caused by a depressive illness rather than an organic dementia. Older people suffering with depression can present in this way. Subjective reports of cognitive impairment may be discrepant with more mild objective findings. The patient may not report any classic features of depression and may not even be aware of being depressed. Objective signs on MSE and MMSE®-2™ as well as clues from the history which point to depression are essential in making this diagnosis. The pattern of memory impairment in pseudodementia is not one that fits with established pathological mechanisms of the dementias. A six-month history of memory loss would, if due to a true dementia, represent an early stage of the disease. At this stage, poor concentration and inattention would be unusual. Depression, however, can impair concentration. The death of her husband was long enough ago that it would be reasonable to assume it is no longer the most direct determinant of her mood.

Poor sleep (C) can be a finding of depression, but is too non-specific and could arise in early dementia when insight is intact and the patient may be anxious about this.

Within six months of a true dementia it would be unlikely for STM and LTM to be so severely affected (D). This in itself, however, is not reliable, as more rare and malignant dementias can cause a rapid progression of cognitive impairment, which would require further testing and investigation.

Weight loss (E) in a 77-year-old with memory impairment could be due to functional impairment and loss of independently managing her activities of daily living (ADL). Of course, physical causes of weight loss should be considered.

18. B ★★★★   OHPsych 3rd edn → pp.89–90, 96

The answer is Cotard syndrome (B), a nihilistic delusion which can arise in severe, psychotic depression, particularly in the elderly. The patient may believe they are already dead, that they do not exist, or that their internal organs are rotting inside them. Mood-congruent delusions are delusions that have a strong affective (mood) component and which are in keeping with the person's prevailing mood. In depression, such a delusion would typically be of content that holds negative views about the person, the world, or the future. In mania, mood-congruent delusions will be of a more grandiose, positive content. Note that mood-incongruent delusions can also arise in both mood disorders and primary psychotic disorders such as schizophrenia.

Capgras syndrome (A) is a delusion of misidentification, thinking somebody familiar has been replaced by an imposter.

Couvade syndrome (C) is a conversion disorder, not a delusion, which arises in partners of pregnant women. The partner begins to experience symptoms of pregnancy such as morning sickness or abdominal discomfort.

Another delusion of misidentification is Frégoli syndrome (D). In this instance the patient believes that a stranger has been replaced by someone familiar.

Othello syndrome (E) is delusional jealousy, where the patient has delusions of their partner's infidelity. Typically this may occur in longstanding alcohol dependence or psychotic disorders such as schizophrenia. The belief can predispose the patient's partner to significant risk of harm.

19. E ★★★   OHpsych 3rd edn → p.72

Perseveration (E) is the most specific frontal lobe sign (and has been described by some as the only pathognomic sign in psychiatry). It may be present in speech or in motor behaviours.

Mild frontal lobe abnormalities constitute part of the natural history of chronic schizophrenia. Frontal lobe abnormalities include reduced volume of prefrontal lobes, although more recent evidence points to pathological changes in connectivity between frontal and temporal lobes. These can also predispose people to developing schizophrenia. Such abnormalities are present in first-episode patients and relatives of people with schizophrenia, indicating a neurodevelopmental mechanism in schizophrenia. Individual frontal lobe signs such as apathy or emotional indifference are often non-specific and must be interpreted in the context of other clinical findings. Apathy (A) can be a sign of frontal lobe damage but can also be a negative symptom of chronic schizophrenia.

Concrete thinking (B) demonstrates an inability to think in abstract terms, and can be tested by asking the patient to interpret a well-known proverb. It is a feature of schizophrenia and can also arise as a result of frontal lobe pathology.

Disinhibition (C) is also a sign of frontal lobe damage, usually involving the orbitofrontal cortex which regulates social behaviour. Disinhibition can also present in acute psychosis and mania.

Inattention (D), another possible frontal lobe sign, can arise in a range of disorders. For instance, in schizophrenia it may represent an onset of auditory hallucinations which prevent the patient from focusing on the interview.

20. E ★★★★   OHPsych 3rd edn → pp.132–3

The answer is inattention (E). Attention is usually preserved in the early stages of cortical dementias.

Amnesia (A) is not the correct answer. Cortical dementias (e.g. Alzheimer's, by far the commonest type) and subcortical dementias (e.g. vascular, Huntington's) have distinct clinical features and time courses, though the precise clinical features depend on the type of dementia, the precise brain parts affected, and the time since onset. A one-year history would be a relatively early stage in Alzheimer's dementia. Memory can be impaired in either type, but is more prominent in cortical dementias.

Aphasias (B) arise if the language centres in Broca's (frontal) or Wernicke's (temporal) areas are affected—these are cortical areas.

Apraxia (C) is usually a feature of cortical dementias affecting the parietal lobe.

Vascular dementia often causes apathy and affective blunting, which can present similarly to depression (D). In the early stage of Alzheimer's dementia, when insight is usually preserved, a reactive depression may also arise.

Extended Matching Questions

1. A ★

A delusional mood is where a person has a sense of something significant about to happen, creating a feeling of perplexity in the patient. It may arise in the prodromal stage of schizophrenia and may precede the onset of more clear-cut systematized delusions. This is otherwise known as delusional atmosphere.

2. I ★

In partition delusions there is the belief that an agent is able to penetrate barriers such as doors, walls, or windows—usually with some sinister purpose. They are more commonly found in older people with new-onset schizophrenia ('paraphrenia').

3. G ★

In nihilistic delusions the person believes that part or all of their body has died. It usually occurs in severe depression and is therefore a mood-congruent delusion. It is otherwise eponymously known as Cotard's delusion.

4. H ★

In psychiatry the term paranoia describes a belief that is self-referential in some way. Note this does not necessarily have to be in a distressing or sinister context, and it is therefore slightly different to the colloquial meaning of paranoia. The paranoid delusion described here is an idea of reference.

5. J ★

Persecutory delusions are usually self-referential (and therefore technically a type of paranoid belief) where the person believes an agent is intentionally trying to harm them in some way. In this case, this is the primary focus, rather than the belief that they are ill, so hypochondriacal delusional would be inaccurate.

→ Johnstone E, Lawrie S, Owens D, and Sharpe MD (2004). *Companion to Psychiatric Studies*, 7th edn. Churchill Livingstone, London.

→ Sims A (2002). *Symptoms in the Mind: An Introduction to Descriptive Psychopathology*, 3rd edn. Saunders, Philadelphia.

General feedback on 1–5: OHPsych 3rd edn → pp.90–2

6. G ★

There is an adequate amount of speech to convey an appropriate response, yet the content contains little meaningful information. This should be distinguished from poverty of speech, where there is a reduced amount of speech and little spontaneity.

7. A ★

In circumstantiality speech is long-winded and difficult to follow, yet still manages to remain focused on the topic of the question. An example from Wikipedia: Q: 'What is your name?' A: 'Well, sometimes when people ask me that I have to think about whether or not I will answer, because some people think it's an odd name, even though I don't really because my mum gave it to me and I think my dad helped, but it's as good a name as any in my opinion. I think it's a little weird to have the same name as two of my other names, but the fact that I like it is a good thing…but yeah, it's Gordon.'

8. C ★

In derailment there is at most only a vague connection between topics. It can be considered to lie on the more extreme end of the spectrum of disconnected thoughts to flight of ideas, in which there is a more clear-cut yet rapid leap from one topic to another. It is typically found in manic or psychotic states. A more extreme disconnect in the speech can cause word salad, in which there is no apparent meaningful/grammatical connection between words.

9. I ★

In tangentiality the patient replies to a question in an oblique manner. As their speech goes on, there is a definite yet highly tenuous connection between topics; there is loss of focus of the original goal of the conversation.

10. B ★

In clanging, the use of words is determined by their sound. Patients' speech may contain a lot of rhyming, alliteration, or punning. It may arise in schizophrenia or other psychotic states.

→ Sims A (2003). *Symptoms in the Mind: An Introduction to Descriptive Psychopathology*, 3rd edn. Saunders, Philadelphia.

General feedback on 6–10: OHPsych 3rd edn → p.96

Assessment and interviewing skills

Susannah Fairweather

Psychiatry is unique as a specialty. In the past century, medical technology has advanced at breakneck speed supporting diagnostic refinement, yet this has had limited impact in the area of mental health. It is not possible to diagnose mental illness with a blood test, a radiological investigation, or other such investigative tools. It requires a doctor to hone their 'end of the bed' observation skills and develop a sophisticated understanding of psychopathology. This familiarity of descriptive psychopathology then needs to be applied in everyday practice to recognize the symptoms being presented, allowing interpretation of illness states. Similar symptoms can present in different illnesses and their relevance needs to be understood in the context of the history of the person. Psychiatric assessments with well-developed interview skills are the cornerstone of psychiatric practice. This can feel a daunting task to medical students and junior doctors who are well used to the protection of many investigation options at their fingertips.

Psychiatric patients are often the most challenging to interview. They can present in ways that confront even the most experienced doctor—highly distressed, aggressive, withdrawn, disconnected from reality, or uncooperative, to describe just a few situations. They may not have chosen to see a doctor and may have come willingly or unwillingly due to someone else's worry about them. These factors often create a difficult starting point from which to engage patients and establish a trusting doctor–patient relationship.

The reasons for a person's presentation, especially in the acute setting, are often highly anxiety provoking—attempted suicide, threatened suicide, or highly disturbed behaviour. This challenges doctors to remain calm in order to maintain the capacity to manage the assessment without relying on the armoury of procedures other specialties often can. A firm grasp of the MSE and the core aspects of a psychiatric history helps to negotiate numerous potential challenges during the interview.

Interviewing and interpretative skills can be developed, akin to a cardiologist learning the sounds of different heart murmurs. The psychiatrist recognizes the increased sounds and behaviours of a manic presentation and the absence of these in depression. Different questioning techniques draw out additional pieces of information, as percussion may further information gathered from auscultation.

The use of the self (or subjective experience) is very important in psychiatric assessment—perhaps a challenge in this evidence-based medicine era. A doctor must notice what it feels like to be in the presence of that person: do they feel sympathy, confused, or buoyed along with the way a person interacts with them? Are they provoked to respond in a certain manner? All of this adds to the deepening understanding of why that person is sitting in front of them at that time and what they may be experiencing.

The family and social context of a presentation are essential, and often requires a wider examination than in other medical presentations. Information may need to be gathered from many sources to piece together a coherent narrative and consequent diagnosis.

Susannah Fairweather

Single Best Answers

QUESTIONS

Single Best Answers

1. A 19-year-old man is accompanied to the ED with two of his friends. He has been hearing sounds and voices and seeing things around him for the last 12 hours. He is in a good mood but a little perplexed. His friends are very worried. Which is the *single* most appropriate initial investigation to determine the cause? ★

A EEG

B Full blood count (FBC)

C Magnetic resonance imaging (MRI) scan of the brain

D Temperature

E Urine drug screen (UDS)

2. A 28-year-old man was found walking along a motorway at 2 am and refused to cooperate with the police interview. The police are concerned that he is a risk to himself and accompany him to the ED. Which is the *single* most important area of assessment to focus on to establish his risk? ★

A Developmental history

B Drug and alcohol history

C Past medical history

D Past psychiatric history

E Thoughts of self-harm or suicide

3. A 21-year-old woman with a longstanding eating disorder attends the day hospital reporting she is not feeling well. Which is the *single* most appropriate physical health parameter to determine her risk at that time? ★

A Heart rate

B Muscular weakness

C Parotid gland enlargement

D Russell's sign

E Weight loss

4. A 54-year-old man requests an alcohol service referral prompted by concerns from his wife after she found him drinking vodka before work to 'settle his nerves'. He says that he knows this is harmful alcohol use but denies he is dependent. Which is the *single* most appropriate area to focus on to clarify his diagnosis? ★

A Frequency of alcohol drinking

B Increased tolerance to alcohol

C Sickness record

D Units of alcohol drunk per week

E Withdrawal symptoms

5. A 32-year-old man has been brought to his general practitioner (GP) by his sister. She worries that he has changed over recent weeks. He has become increasingly preoccupied with being the son of Zeus and sharing this with others. His clothes have become more flamboyant. He is particularly noisy at night which is causing problems with his neighbours. He is singing loudly to the waiting room as he waits to be seen. Which is the *single* most appropriate aspect of sleep to focus on during the assessment to help formulate a diagnosis? ★

A Duration of sleep

B Presence of dreams

C Presence of sleep-walking

D Quality of sleep

E Sleep-onset difficulties

6. A 22-year-old woman has low mood and is missing work. She has superficial scars on her forearms. She is quite guarded about suicidal thoughts and denies any plans. Her partner found a pro-suicide website open on her computer. She is known to be a frequent Twitter user. Which is the *single* most appropriate assessment action regarding her social media use? ★

A Ask her next of kin to find out what is on her account

B Contact Twitter administration to request her account details

C Ignore her Twitter account

D Look up her public profile

E Send her a follower request

7. A 35-year-old man took an overdose of four 500 mg paracetamol tablets over two hours alone in his flat. He states he did it with the intention to die. Which is the *single* most appropriate indicator to assess the risk of the overdose? ★

A Amount of paracetamol taken

B Intention of overdose

C Overdose taken alone in flat

D Physical effects of overdose

E Way in which the overdose was taken, i.e. staggered over time

8. A 42-year-old woman is on a neurology ward. She has undergone extensive investigation for a right leg paralysis, with no underlying organic cause found. She is able to answer questions clearly, concisely, and accurately. She is calm and accepting of her situation. Which is the *single* most appropriate description of this mental state abnormality? ★

A Disorientation

B Mood incongruence

C Perceptual abnormalities

D Speech abnormality

E Thought disorder

9. A 72-year-old recent widower attends his GP reporting a history of low mood, tearfulness, episodes of agitation, and no hope for the future. He believes he is depressed and would like antidepressant medication. Which is the *single* most appropriate area to focus on to clarify this diagnosis? ★

A ADL

B Bereavement history

C Change in appetite

D Previous history of similar episodes

E Sleep pattern changes

10. A 32-year-old woman is brought to the ED by police. She was observed behaving as though she was planning to jump off a local bridge. This is her twelfth presentation related to suicide in the last two months. The ED staff make derogatory comments about her to the psychiatrist and appear unsympathetic. Which is the *single* most appropriate diagnosis? ★

A Anxious personality disorder (PD)

B Borderline PD

C Dissocial PD

D Histrionic PD

E Narcissistic PD

11. A 17-year-old adolescent is brought to the ED by the police. He became aggressive while at a local youth centre and damaged property. A psychiatric review is requested from ED staff. Before agreeing to this, he says that he is does not want anybody else to be told anything about what he says in the interview. Which is the *single* most appropriate reason for his confidentiality to be breached? ★★

A Parental request as they claim parental right to know

B Police request to support their investigation

C Report from him of a risk to himself or others

D Social services request to help triage the referral about him sent to them

E Youth centre's request for information to help their understanding of the incident

12. A 24-year-old man has always felt, from a very young age, that he was female. He has always been attracted to males. He has worn women's clothing since puberty, wears make-up, waxes excess hair from his body, and grows his hair long. This has been accepted by his friends and family. He feels a lot of distress about not having the physical characteristics of a woman. Which is the *single* most likely diagnosis? ★★

A Homosexuality

B Multiple disorders of sexual preference

C Paedophilia

D Transsexualism

E Transvestism

13. An eight-year-old boy was referred by his school due to their concerns that he tends to be alone in the playground at break times and has no friends. He struggles with any changes. They note he seems to only eat cornflakes. He cannot tie his shoelaces and has poor handwriting. Which is the *single* most appropriate area of developmental history to focus on to determine diagnosis? ★★

A Feeding history

B Medical history

C Motor development history

D Pregnancy history

E Social communication history

14. A 27-year-old woman is admitted following a suicide attempt. She is already under the care of a mental health team. She tells the duty psychiatrist that she has never felt so understood before, feels much better following her assessment, and, because of this, would like to remain in touch with her. She suggests meeting the following week in the hospital canteen to report back on her progress. Which is the *single* most appropriate course of action for the duty doctor to follow? ★★

A Clearly explain that the duty doctor will not be able to meet independently and that the patient's team will review her progress

B Contact the patient's care coordinator to discuss the request and get their opinion on whether it is a good idea

C Inform ward nursing staff about the request and ask them to manage the situation without involving the duty doctor

D Plan a time to meet her in a clinical area the following week to review her progress

E Provide a bleep number in order to support the patient during her admission and arrange a meeting to review

15. A 17-year-old adolescent is brought to the ED by police under a Section 136 of the MHA 1983. The police had been requested to attend her college following her becoming agitated and damaging property. It is not clear why the episode occurred. Which is the *single* most appropriate reason for her confidentiality being breached without her consent? ★★

A College staff request to support their investigation and disciplinary procedures

B Individual report of on-going risk to self and others

C Insurance company request to process the claim made by the college

D Parental request to understand events and support their daughter

E Police request as part of their criminal investigation against her

16. A 16-year-old adolescent says she was taught about experiments in her psychology lesson that day. She believes this occurred because she is part of a secret experiment and 'they' are letting her know about it. Which is the *single* most appropriate description of the delusion she is experiencing? ★★★

A Autochthonous delusion

B Delusional atmosphere

C Delusional memory

D Delusional percept

E Grandiose delusion

17. A 23-year-old woman sees her GP as she is concerned about seeing blood in her vomit. After starting university she began to vomit after eating to reduce her weight. She describes never feeling so good about her current weight and getting many compliments about her slim figure. She found the transition to university difficult in part due to low self-esteem, having been bullied from a young age due to being overweight. Which is the *single* most accurate description of the maintaining factor for her behaviour? ★★★

A Concern about blood in her vomit

B Feeling good about her current weight

C History of bullying

D Slim figure

E Struggling with move to university

18. A 21-year-old man comes to the ED and says he has 'brain fag' and needs urgent help. The ED doctor is baffled. Which is the *single* most appropriate area of assessment to focus on to understand the self diagnosis? ★★★

A Cultural background

B Drug and alcohol history

C Education history

D Precipitating events to presentation

E Social history

19. A seven-year-old boy is referred for assessment by his school. He is reported to be doing poorly in class despite being thought to be academically able. He fidgets a lot, seems unable to sit as long as the other children, often blurts out answers, and appears to daydream. Which is the *single* most appropriate tool to administer prior to him attending clinic? ★★★★

A Children's Global Assessment Scale (CGAS)

B Conners' Rating Scale

C Health of the Nation Outcome Scales for Children and Adolescents (HoNOSCA)

D Mood and Feelings Questionnaire (MFQ)

E Strengths and Difficulties Questionnaire (SDQ)

20. A family have on-going difficulties in their relationships. There is a concern that conflict within the family is worsening the father's chronic mental health difficulties. They have been referred for an assessment of suitability for family therapy. Which is the *single* most likely form of questioning to be used in this situation? ★★★★

A Circular questioning

B Direct questions

C Motivational questioning

D Open questions

E Socratic questioning

Extended Matching Questions

Anxiety disorders

For each scenario below, choose the *single* most likely diagnosis from the list of options. Each option may be used once, more than once, or not at all. ★

A Acute stress reaction

B Adjustment disorder

C Agoraphobia

D Claustrophobia

E Generalized anxiety disorder

F Obsessive-compulsive disorder (OCD)

G Panic disorder

H PTSD

I Separation anxiety

J Social phobia

1. A 45-year-old man keeps worrying something bad is going to happen to his wife and children. He has developed a pattern of checking all the windows and doors in his house five times before he settles to bed at night.

2. A five-year-old boy has found it difficult to settle into school for six months. His mother continues to stay in the classroom because, when she tries to leave, he becomes very distressed, crying and struggling to breathe. He has never been able to go to a friend's house to play without her present.

3. A 28-year-old woman is admitted to an orthopaedic ward with a broken leg and pelvis following a road traffic collision (RTC) last night. She is dazed and confused. She feels her heart is 'beating too fast' and feels extremely anxious when her family leaves her.

4. A 52-year-old woman struggles to leave her house, buys all her shopping online, and has lost contact with her local community. She has not travelled on a bus or the London Underground for three years because she gets too worried that she may be trapped in a situation she can't easily escape from.

5. A 22-year-old man feels very lonely despite having a successful university career. He struggles to accept any social invitations from other students. He is particularly concerned that he has a tendency to blush and a constant need to go to the toilet in these situations.

Speech disorders

For each scenario below, choose the *single* most appropriate type of speech or thought disorder from the list of options. Each option may be used once, more than once, or not at all. ★

A Circumstantiality

B Derailment

C Echolalia

D Flight of ideas

E Knight's move thinking

F Perseveration

G Tangentiality

H Thought blocking

I Thought insertion

J Word salad

6. A 67-year-old man is assessed in the ED. When asked his name he responds 'John'. When asked why he is in the hospital today he responds 'John'. When asked what is wrong, the man responds 'John'.

7. A 25-year-old man spends 10 minutes explaining in great detail his journey to get to the clinic when asked how his journey was to get to clinic.

8. A six-year-old boy responds 'play with jigsaw' when asked 'Would you like to play with the jigsaw?'

9. A 19-year-old woman feels that her mind is being altered. She says she knows it's due to aliens making her think things that they want her to think.

10. A 35-year-old woman starts talking about buying new swim-wear, her holiday plans, and her plan to set up a new travel company, after the receptionist comments on the lovely weather. She talks too quickly for the receptionist to interrupt.

ANSWERS

Single Best Answers

1. E ★   OHPsych 3rd edn → pp.130–1

Given the short duration of the presentation and the multiperceptual nature of his symptoms, it is likely these are drug-induced symptoms. UDS (E) can be found in most ED, but may have to be specially requested, as it is not commonly used outside of psychiatric assessments.

Sensory disturbance can be a symptom of epilepsy; however, it is likely there would be other symptoms suggesting epilepsy and the need for an EEG (A).

An FBC would be useful to assess for an infective cause of his presentation, ruling out a delirium; however, his good mood would suggest against delirium (B).

Whilst visual hallucinations can be part of an organic presentation, the MRI scan would not be a first-line investigation (C). The short duration of symptoms would suggest a different cause.

A temperature (D) would be a useful investigation to rule out a possible infection. Some illicit drugs such as ecstasy, which has the active component 3,4-methylenedioxy-N-methylamphetamine (MDMA), are also known to raise temperature. However, the result would not differentiate between diagnoses.

→ RCPsych information for young people on drugs and alcohol: http://www.rcpsych.ac.uk/healthadvice/parentsandyouthinfo/youngpeople/drugsandalcohol.aspx.

→ RCPsych information on psychosis for parents, carers and anyone who works with young people: http://www.rcpsych.ac.uk/healthadvice/parentsandyouthinfo/parentscarers/psychosis.aspx.

2. E ★   OHPsych 3rd edn → p.52

In order to establish the risk at the point of assessment, direct assessment needs to establish whether the individual has thoughts of self-harm and suicide (E), the intention they have regarding this, and whether any plans have been formulated. In the past mental health staff have been concerned that by asking directly about self-harm and suicide, it may prompt an individual to have such thoughts. It is widely agreed this view is inaccurate and that specific assessment needs to occur in every assessment.

A developmental history (A) will focus on the early development of an individual, such as their speech and language and motor development. This is important to know about as it may contribute to any risks posed by the man to himself or others. However, it will not help establish immediate risk.

Drug and alcohol use are known to increase risk for people in terms of risk to both self and others, due to their effect on functioning and mental state. Drug and alcohol history alone will not identify immediate risk for an individual (B).

Past medical history (C) can contribute to risk, for example if the individual has a chronic illness or terminal illness. This part of the history would give an idea of contributing factors to risk but not establish the immediate risk for an individual.

Past psychiatric history (D) is very important in supporting understanding the level of risk in an individual. It is well established that if an individual has harmed themselves, has a history of suicide attempts, or has a history of harm to others there is a higher likelihood of this occurring again. If an individual has an established psychiatric diagnosis this will also raise their level of risk. However this will not identify the immediate risk at the point of assessment.

→ Centre for Suicide Research, Department of Psychiatry, University of Oxford, Assessment of suicide risk in people with depression, a clinical guide: http://cebmh.warne.ox.ac.uk/csr/Clinical_guide_assessing_suicide_risk.pdf

3. A ★   OHPsych 3rd edn → pp.400–3

Heart rate (A) is the physical parameter with the most immediate impact on risk. Ideally it should be interpreted with blood pressure. Women with chronic low weight are likely to have chronic bradycardia, but a heart rate of less than 50 beats per minute (bpm) is extremely concerning. It is also advisable that an ECG is carried out.

Muscular weakness (B) is a sign of severity of malnutrition. It is most commonly assessed by the sit-up, squat–stand test. This assesses the ability of an individual to sit up from lying and to stand from squatting, rating it depending on ability and need to use arms for assistance. Whilst it is very important to assess, it is not the best indicator for immediate physical risk.

Parotid gland enlargement (C) is a sign of repeated vomiting. It is a concerning sign but not one that would alter immediate physical management.

Russell's sign (D) is a sign defined by calluses on the knuckles or back of the hand due to repeated self-induced vomiting over long periods of time. Its presence does not affect immediate physical risk.

Weight loss (E) is a very important physical parameter, especially if weight loss has occurred in a large amount over a short period of time in an already underweight individual. However, weight loss alone would not determine immediate physical health management.

→ RCPsych MARSIPAN: Management of really sick patients with anorexia nervosa: http://www.rcpsych.ac.uk/publications/collegereports/cr/cr162.aspx.

4. E ★   OHPsych 3rd edn → p.542

Dependency syndrome is a cluster of behavioural, cognitive, and physiological phenomena that develop after repeated substance use and which typically include a strong desire to drink alcohol, difficulties in controlling its use, persisting in its use despite harmful consequences, a higher priority given to drinking alcohol than to other activities and obligations, increased tolerance, and sometimes a physical withdrawal state. The presence of withdrawal symptoms shows physical dependency and therefore is the best way to determine between simple harmful alcohol use and true dependency (E).

The frequency of drinking alcohol (A) may suggest harmful drinking patterns as well as dependency. It is necessary to consider how often but also when drinking takes place.

Increased tolerance to alcohol (B) is likely to be present in both harmful and dependent drinking. Also the type of alcohol consumed can alert you to increased tolerance, as often lager/cider drinkers will shift to spirits as their tolerance increases to avoid drinking excessive quantities of liquid.

A change in sickness record (C) could be present in both harmful and dependent drinking. The nature of the work should be considered in detail, as there are legal and professional obligations to alert governing bodies in relation to certain jobs, for example lorry drivers.

Information on amounts of alcohol ingested and associated risks would not determine between harmful use and dependency. High amounts of units of alcohol drunk per week (D) will impact on treatment, as there will be an increased risk of serious withdrawal effects as well as chronic complications.

→ RCPsych information on alcohol use: http://www.rcpsych.ac.uk/ mentalhealthinfoforall/problems/alcoholanddrugs/alcoholourfavourit-edrug.aspx.

5. A ★   OHPsych 3rd edn → pp.306, 420–2

This man is presenting with symptoms suggestive of a manic presentation. The typical sleep pattern associated with this is to have minimal sleep or none at all, due to a feeling of extreme energy. Therefore asking about duration of sleep (A) is the most appropriate approach to help make a diagnosis.

The presence of dreams (B) is not associated with psychopathology or mental illness.

The presence of sleep-walking (C) is not associated with psychopathology or mental illness. Also known as somnambulism, it is most common in children with the peak age at six years (around 20% of all four to eight year olds). However, in a recently published study about 4% of American adults reported two or more episodes of sleep-walking per month.

Poor quality sleep (D) and sleep-onset difficulties (E) are more associated with depression and anxiety states than hypomanic/manic states.

→ RCPsych information on bipolar disorder which includes a section on mania: http://www.rcpsych.ac.uk/mentalhealthinfo/problems/bipolardisorder/bipolardisorder.aspx.

6. D ★   OHPsych 3rd edn → p.898

The answer is to look up her public profile (D). There is a legitimate reason to gather collateral information regarding the risk presented by this patient. She is guarded, but there is evidence to suggest she is contemplating further, more serious self-harm, and her management plan should take this into account. In this case, it would seem fair to assume that the Twitter account will help provide appropriate collateral information regarding her state of mind. There is no question that attempting to access private sites, such as 'protected tweets', through honest or dishonest means is considered unethical and inappropriate, in much the same way as breaking into someone's house to find out how they really live would be clearly wrong. Ethics experts advise that accessing public profiles isn't necessarily wrong or unethical, as long as the healthcare professional keeps the patient's best interests in mind. Tweets should not be read to add excitement or gossip into the consultation but to gain an understanding of the risks.

Asking her next of kin to find out what is on her account is not the answer (A). It is not the responsibility of the next of kin to spy on the patient or to act on the doctor's behalf to uncover information at their request. It would be ethical and appropriate to ask the next of kin for their opinion about the patient's risks and to gather collateral from them about any previous significant events. It would also be fair to ask them about the use of Twitter in relation to the patient's mental health (i.e. does it make it better or worse?).

Contacting Twitter administration to request her account details is both inappropriate and dangerous (B). As a doctor, you have no right to request this information (it would need to be the police or Home Office in relation to a serious threat), but also the time taken for the request and its information would delay managing her care appropriately while waiting for it.

As her use of Twitter was brought up during an appropriate assessment it would be wrong to ignore it (C). In every history it is sensible to consider online use and possible stressors, including bullying (school and workplace), dangerous behaviours, and sexual risk, as well as protective factors such as support networks, healthy outlets of emotion, and help-seeking behaviours. Increasingly, the online world inhabited by a patient is an important area to consider when assessing them and planning their treatment.

Sending her a follower request would not be appropriate as it would be considered a blurring of professional and personal boundaries (E). The advice of the RCPsych is to 'adopt the simplest approach to social media…completely separate personal social media sites from professional ones, and to have the highest level of privacy in place on personal sites'. We should be aware of what we are posting on Twitter, Facebook, Tumblr, Instagram, etc. and keep aware of changes to the General Medical Council's (GMC's) Good Medical Practice regarding social media use.

→ RCPsych leaflet 'On professional boundaries': http://www.rcpsych. ac.uk/pdf/18%20on%20boundaries_final.pdf.

→ Wuyts P, Broome M, and McGuire P (2011). Assessing the mental state through a blog: psychiatry in the 21st century? *The Psychiatrist*, **35**, 361–3.

7. B ★   OHPsych 3rd edn → pp.784–7

The man stated he took the overdose with the intention to die. Although the clinician knows the overdose would not be lethal, the patient's intention suggested he believed it would be. Therefore this is the best predictor of his risk (B).

The amount of paracetamol taken (A) by the man was small. Therefore if one is to judge risk by this indicator, his risk would be thought to be low. However, some people may not be aware of what doses of medication would be lethal in overdose, and thus it is not useful to assess risk by amount of substance taken.

The risk of an overdose taken by someone alone does suggest the possibility of a higher risk, but it is not the best predicator of risk in this scenario (C).

The physical effect of this overdose (D) is likely to be negligible. If risk is based on this, his risk would be deemed low. However, it is important to take seriously what a person says in their history, rather than assuming anything from the result of their actions.

A staggered overdose of paracetamol (E) has the potential to be more damaging. However, a staggered overdose on its own may not indicate the level of risk and therefore it is not the best indicator of risk in this scenario.

→ NICE Clinical Guideline 16— Self-harm: the short-term physical and psychological management and secondary prevention of self-harm in primary and secondary care: http://www.nice.org.uk/nicemedia/live/10946/29421/29421.pdf.

8. B ★   OHPsych 3rd edn → pp.56–7, 64–5

The answer is mood incongruence (B). The history suggests she is presenting with a dissociative paralysis of her right leg because no organic cause has been found. This is more commonly seen in women than men and was previously known as hysteria. It is now more commonly termed under 'medically unexplained symptoms' (MUS). On MSE there is often little abnormality. The classic finding is that mood is often incongruent to the level of disability the person is experiencing. It is referred to as 'belle indifference' as the person is unexpectedly calm and accepting of the disability.

She appears to be orientated in time, place, and person. This is a useful test of orientation, although common sense should be used, for example if a patient has been admitted overnight they may get the day wrong or not know exactly where they are. Asking for a birthday or home address is not a test for disorientation (A) as these memories are stored in long-term memory.

She is not reporting any perceptual abnormalities (C) such as seeing something that is not there or hearing sounds that nobody else is aware of. In general, perceptual abnormalities may not always be fully formed and therefore may be reported as 'shadows' or 'noises'—called elemental abnormalities.

She is able to answer questions without any apparent problem. When considering speech abnormalities (D), it is important to differentiate between expressive problems, where there is a problem forming and articulating the words, and receptive problems, where the patient's communication is hindered by their inability to organize their words, resulting in meaningless language.

A formal thought disorder (E) would be seen as disorganized speech as a result of disorganized thinking, as seen most commonly in psychosis. There would usually be a degree of distress associated with this as the patient becomes increasingly upset and annoyed.

→ Functional and dissociative neurological symptoms: a patient's guide: http://www.neurosymptoms.org/.

9. B ★   OHPsych 3rd edn → pp.520–1

The answer is bereavement history (B). The diagnosis needs to be considered within the context of this man being a 'recent widower'. The symptoms he describes to the GP could be part of a normal bereavement reaction if they are occurring weeks to months after his partner's death, or they could be symptoms of a depressive episode if the bereavement occurred a longer time ago.

ADLs (A) are often affected in many psychiatric illnesses and as part of a normal bereavement response. This does not allow differentiation of a diagnosis.

A change in appetite (C) is a symptom that occurs in many different psychiatric presentations and is not limited to one diagnosis.

Previous similar episodes will give an indication of past psychiatric history, but this will not allow differentiation of diagnosis (D).

An alteration in sleep pattern (E) is a common symptom in a wide range of psychiatric illnesses and normal experiences. Therefore it is neither diagnostic nor specific enough to allow a differentiation of diagnosis.

→ RCPsych information on depression in older adults: http://www.rcpsych.ac.uk/mentalhealthinfoforall/problems/depression/depressioninolderadults.aspx.

→ RCPsych information on bereavement: http://www.rcpsych.ac.uk/mentalhealthinfoforall/problems/bereavement/bereavement.aspx.

10. B ★   OHPsych 3rd edn → pp.504–5

The answer is borderline PD (B) (of which this is the emotionally unstable subtype) is characterized by a definite tendency to act impulsively and without consideration of the consequences. The person's mood is often unpredictable and they are liable to outbursts of emotion and an incapacity to control their behavioural explosions. They can often present with self-destructive behaviours, including suicide gestures and attempts. People with this PD often provoke strong feelings from healthcare professionals looking after them.

Anxious PD (A) is characterized by feelings of tension and apprehension, insecurity, and inferiority. There is a continuous yearning to be liked and accepted, a hypersensitivity to rejection and criticism with restricted personal attachments, and a tendency to avoid certain activities by habitual exaggeration of the potential dangers or risks in everyday situations. It is neither characteristic for people with this to repeatedly present to EDs nor to repeatedly act in a risky manner related to suicide.

Dissocial PD (C) is characterized by disregard for social obligations and callous unconcern for the feelings of others. The person can often display violence. They may present to EDs frequently due to injuries sustained from violence, but this is not common. They are often well known in the criminal justice system. They do not normally present with repeated suicidal acts.

Histrionic PD (D) is characterized by shallow and labile affect, self-dramatization, theatricality, exaggerated expression of emotions, suggestibility, egocentricity, self-indulgence, lack of consideration for others, easily hurt feelings, and continuous seeking for appreciation, excitement, and attention. There is not a tendency to engage in repeated suicidal attempts or gestures, nor does the person present frequently to EDs.

Narcissistic PD (E) is characterized by an inflated sense of self-importance and an extreme preoccupation with oneself. There is neither a tendency to act out in dramatic ways nor to present with repeated suicide attempts or gestures. The person does not commonly present repeatedly to emergency services.

→ RCPsych information on personality disorder: http://www.rcpsych. ac.uk/expertadvice/problems/personalitydisorders/personalitydisorder.aspx.

→ NICE Clinical Guideline 78—Borderline personality disorder: http:// www.nice.org.uk/CG78.

11. C ★★   OHPsych 3rd edn → pp.898–901

The answer is (C). If any medical professional is concerned about a significant risk to an individual or that the individual poses a significant risk to others, medical confidentiality can be breached. It is the duty of the healthcare professional to either pass this information on to the appropriate authority or to seek help to find out who that might be. It is best practice to inform the patient before doing this unless it will increase the danger.

Parental request as they claim parental 'right' to know is also the wrong answer (A). There is strict guidance on when medical confidentiality can be breached. The scenario is made slightly more complex given that the adolescent is 17 years old. However, at the age of 16 an adolescent is thought to have capacity (Mental Capacity Act, 2005). Therefore, parents do not have a right to know anything she discloses without her consent.

There is no obligation for a medical professional to breach confidentiality to a place of education or the police (B) unless dictated by law or social services and there are significant safeguarding concerns.

Social services' request to help triage the referral about him sent to them (D) is not a reason to breach confidentiality. The referral should consider the risk presented by the patient and what information they need to know to work with him. A clear summary of the situation should be given, preferably with the agreement of the patient beforehand, and not as a response to a triage request.

The centre's request for information to help their understanding of the incident is not the answer (E). There is no legal obligation to do this. It would be helpful to consider the act with the patient and to take this into account in his management, plus a conversation could be had with the youth centre about their general policies, but this should not include any specific disclosures.

→ General Medical Council guidance on confidentiality: http://www. gmc-uk.org/guidance/ethical_guidance/confidentiality.asp.

12. D ★★   OHPsych 3rd edn → pp.484–7

This man is clearly describing transsexualism (D). He has a desire to live and be accepted as a member of the opposite sex by dressing as a female, which is accompanied by a sense of discomfort with his own anatomic sex.

The man reports feeling that he is a woman and from this is attracted to men. Homosexuality (A) is being sexually attracted to members of the same sex and does not include feeling like the opposite sex internally. Homosexuality is not a psychiatric disorder, although in the past it has been classified as such.

There is no suggestion that this man has any disorders of sexual preference (B) as defined in the International Statistical Classification of Diseases and Related Health Problems 10th Revision (ICD-10) (or 'paraphilias in the Diagnostic and Statistical Manual of Mental Disorders Fifth Edition (DSM-V)). Disorders of sexual preference are patterns of sexual behaviour that cause distress or difficulty to the person. ICD-10 gives examples of fetishism, transvestism, and sadomasochism. If these behaviours are considered harmless or conducted by mutually consenting partners they should not be defined as a disorder.

There is no suggestion that this man has a 'persistent or a predominant preference for sexual activity with a prepubescent child or children', the ICD-10 definition of paedophilia (C). He is described as being attracted to males all his life but this is within the developmentally normal context.

Transvestism (E) is the wearing of clothes of the opposite sex principally to obtain sexual excitement and to create the appearance of a person of the opposite sex. Fetishistic transvestism is distinguished from transsexual transvestism by its clear association with sexual arousal and the strong desire to remove the clothing once orgasm occurs and sexual arousal declines. It can occur as an earlier phase in the development of transsexualism. There is no evidence this man is wearing female clothing specifically for sexual excitement; rather it relates to his sense of his gender.

→ NHS choices article on gender identity disorder including a video interview with a woman who changed gender:http://www.nhs.uk/conditions/gender-dysphoria/pages/introduction.aspx.

13. E ★★   OHPsych 3rd edn → pp.630–1

The history is strongly suggestive of social communication difficulties (E), likely ASD, and this requires a thorough assessment of his social communication history.

The scenario suggests the boy may have selective eating; however, this is only part of his difficulties. A feeding history (A) will not provide enough information to make a diagnosis. Feeding and eating difficulties are often part of an autistic spectrum disorder (ASD).

A medical history (B) will be useful but is unlikely to clarify between differential diagnoses.

The boy is reported to have fine motor difficulties as part of his presentation. This is often seen in children with an ASD. A history regarding his motor development (C) is useful but will not be sufficient to assess all the concerns.

The pregnancy history (D) will allow assessment of any trauma or complications in the prenatal period but will not lead to a clear diagnosis with a complete assessment.

→ National Autistic Society: http://www.autism.org.uk/.

→ RCPsych information on autism and Asperger's syndrome: http://www.rcpsych.ac.uk/healthadvice/parentsandyouthinfo/parentscarers/autismandaspergerssyndrome.aspx.

14. A ★★   OHPsych 3rd edn → pp.506–9

Clearly explaining that they will not be able to meet independently and that the patient's team will review her progress is the correct way forward (A). A clear and definitive response given to the patient at the time of the request leaves her with no ambiguity about the potential of further meetings. The situation and outcome should be clearly documented in the patient records in case of future complaints. This scenario is relatively common, especially for junior doctors working in psychiatry for the first time. There are suggestions from the history that the patient may have a PD given that she is well known and admitted a suicide attempt. Her idealization of the duty psychiatrist represents the psychodynamic concept of 'splitting' which often occurs with this type of patient. Professionals providing care often get positioned in either 'good' or 'bad' roles. There are different ways to manage the attempt at achieving a professional boundary violation. The most straightforward way is to deal with it at the time in a clear and polite manner. It is also important to make other professionals involved in her care aware of it either by clear documentation or by discussion. This limits the potential of splitting or allegations being made in the future.

Contacting the patient's care coordinator to discuss the request and get their opinion on whether it is a good idea (B) is not the answer. This will result in no clear decision being communicated to the patient at the time of request and therefore she is left with a hope of the meeting occurring. The duty doctor is acting properly in consulting the appropriate colleague responsible for the patient's care and informing them of the request, but they should not consider fulfilling this.

It would be wrong to inform ward nursing staff about the request and ask them to manage the situation without involving the duty doctor (C). The duty doctor would be correct to inform the nursing staff of the situation, but not to leave it to them to manage, as the request came directly to the doctor and therefore the doctor is responsible for managing it.

Planning a time to meet her in a clinical area the following week to review her progress (D) would constitute a professional boundary violation as the duty doctor has no role in the patient's on-going care. Although a meeting held in a clinical setting, rather than the canteen, upholds confidentiality and will allow for a more professional assessment, in this case the meeting in itself is not appropriate.

Providing a bleep number in order to support the patient during her admission and arranging a meeting to review (E) would constitute a professional boundary violation as the duty doctor has no role in the patient's on-going care. Doctors should be careful about the appropriateness of giving patients a way to contact them directly and should not enter into this without consulting their team and senior colleagues. This may precipitate a situation where the doctor feels solely responsible for a patient's wellbeing even when not on duty.

→ RCPsych information on professional and personal relationships: http://www.rcpsych.ac.uk/discoverpsychiatry/studentassociates/perspective-sonpsychiatry/drawingfromlife/keepingmum/relationship.aspx.

→ RCPsych information on Good Psychiatric Practice: www.rcpsych.ac.uk/files/pdfversion/CR154.pdf.

15. B ★★   OHPsych 3rd edn → pp.900–1

The correct answer is individual report of on-going risk to self and others (B). The GMC provides very specific guidance about situations in which medical confidentiality can be breached without consent. The 17-year-old is deemed to have capacity under the Mental Capacity Act 2005 unless it has been specifically assessed that she does not. However, in order to maintain her safety and/or that of others, information can be shared with appropriate others if she discloses information that is deemed to be significantly risky.

College staff requesting to support their investigation and disciplinary procedures is not a reason to breach confidentiality (A). However, it might be worth considering a letter of support for her that does not disclose the full extent of her mental health issues but could advocate on her behalf.

Insurance company request to process the claim made by the college (C) is a wrong answer. It is the responsibility of the college to deal with their insurance, not the doctor. The duty of care is to the patient not to the college. If she wishes to give her permission for this, then it would be fair to answer the request.

Breaching confidentiality because of parental request to understand events and support their daughter (D) would be wrong. There is no 'right' to have this information, and therefore consent needs to be sought before doing so. However, it would be appropriate to discuss fully with the patient why her parents want to know the information and how they might be supportive of her, which may involve some sharing of information. If she still refuses, and has the capacity to do so, then this must be the guiding decision. In every case, the discussion and outcome should be clearly documented in the notes.

Police request as part of their criminal investigation against her (E) is also a wrong answer. The police can request this information and it would be up to the doctor to discuss the request with the patient and then to fol-low the patient's wishes. If the police disagree with this, then it is up to them to launch a formal request for this via the court system.

→ General Medical Council guidance on confidentiality: http://www.gmc-uk.org/guidance/ethical_guidance/confidentiality.asp.

16. D ★★★   OHPsych 3rd edn → pp.59–61

This is a delusional percept (D). The woman has had an experience and, at that time, interprets this with a delusional meaning. The perceptual experience can be understood in a broad sense related to perceiving both an object and the sense of written or spoken messages in this case.

Autochthonous delusion (A) cannot be correct because the delusion has not come out of the blue but rather follows on 'logically' from an experi-ence the patient has had.

Delusional atmosphere (B) relates to a general atmosphere and not a delusion in response to a perception.

Delusional memory (C) refers to when a patient recalls an event or idea that is clearly delusional; therefore the delusion is retrojected in time. This can be a false memory but is better used as a real memory which is remembered, then given a delusional meaning.

A grandiose delusion (E) refers to the content of the delusion rather than the form. Her delusion is not grandiose in content.

→ Sims A (2002). *Symptoms in the Mind: An Introduction to Descriptive Psychopathology*, 3rd edn, pp.117–48. Saunders, Philadelphia

17. B ★★★   OHPsych 3rd edn → p.46

The answer is feeling good about her current weight (B). A maintaining factor is something that supports a behaviour continuing. The woman reports feeling good about her current weight. If she links this being a result of the vomiting, she is more likely to continue the vomiting. Therefore it is a maintaining factor.

Concern about blood in her vomit (A) is the wrong answer. The woman's concern about the harm her behaviour is causing her physical health has motivated her to seek medical attention. Therefore, it would be thought of as a motivating factor for change rather than a maintaining factor.

The history of bullying (C) about being overweight is a factor that would predispose the woman to seek out weight loss behaviours. The bullying is historical and so is not a maintaining factor currently.

The woman is getting compliments on her slim figure (D) which could be a maintaining factor for continued behaviour. However, a slim figure on its own may not be a maintaining factor.

The stress of starting university (E) and the consequent behaviours to manage this and her weight is a precipitating factor and not a maintaining factor because in the scenario there is no indication this is ongoing.

→ British Psychological Society Good Practice Guidelines on the use of psychological (psychiatric) formulation: http://www.canterbury. ac.uk/social-applied-sciences/ASPD/documents/DCPGuidelinesfor formulation2011.pdf

18. A ★★★   OHPsych 3rd edn → pp.912–14, 916–17

Brain fag is an example of a culture-bound syndrome. It is a term used almost exclusively in West Africa but is becoming slightly more widespread. It is a term meaning mental exhaustion. It is seen predominantly in male students studying for exams. It generally manifests as vague somatic symptoms, depression, and difficulty concentrating. It can be considered an anxiety disorder too. Therefore, understanding the cultural context (A) of the self-diagnosis will be the most useful for the emergency doctor in understanding the presentation.

Brain fag is not a syndrome related to drugs and alcohol, so focusing on this area of history will not support understanding of the self-diagnosis (B).

Brain fag is commonly reported to occur at times of increased academic pressure such as exams. An education history (C) encompasses all of a person's school and university history. It may help to understand if the man has experienced this before during his education but will not help the doctor to understand the self-diagnosis more.

An understanding of the precipitating events (D) will be very useful for the doctor to know the context in which the brain fag has occurred. However, it may not be sufficient to understand what is meant by brain fag.

A social history (E) will be helpful in understanding the man's functioning currently and any other relevant contributing factors. However, it is not as specific as cultural background and may not capture the information needed to understand the context of the self diagnosis.

→ Sims A (2002). *Symptoms in the Mind: An Introduction to Descriptive Psychopathology*, 3rd edn, pp.403–4. Saunders, Philadelphia.

19. B ★★★★   OHPsych 3rd edn → pp.80–2

The Conners' Rating Scale (B) is a specific screening tool for ADHD. The referral is strongly suggestive of a boy with ADHD symptoms and therefore this tool would be the most appropriate to gather information prior to assessment. It is usually given both to parents and the teacher. In older children (or adults) there is a self-report scale.

The CGAS (A) is a numeric scale used by mental health professionals to rate general functioning of children under 18. It is independent of diagnosis. Given that the boy has not yet been seen and it is a very general scale it will not help the clinician prior to assessing him in clinic.

HoNOSCA (C) is a routine outcome measurement tool that assesses the behaviours, impairments, symptoms, and social functioning of children and adolescents with mental health problems. It provides a global measure of an individual's current mental health status, and thus provides a means of evaluating the success of attempts to improve the health and social functioning of mentally ill children and adolescents. Given that this boy has not yet been seen in clinic, it would not be the most appropriate to administer prior to assessment.

MFQ (D) is a 32-item questionnaire based on the diagnostic criteria for depression. It is used for children from age 6–18. It consists of a series of descriptive phrases regarding how the child has been feeling or acting recently. Codings reflect whether the phrase was descriptive of the subject most of the time, sometimes, or not at all in the past two weeks. The referral for the boy may have an emotional component; however, this would not be the first line of assessment and therefore not the most appropriate choice in this case.

SDQ (E) is a brief behavioural screening questionnaire about 3- to 16-year-olds. It assesses the following domains: emotional symptoms, conduct problems, hyperactivity/inattention, peer relationship problems, and prosocial behaviour. It is a very useful tool. However, given the boy's presenting symptoms, it is not the most appropriate tool.

→ NICE Guidance for the diagnosis and management of ADHD: http://www.nice.org.uk/nicemedia/live/12061/42060/42060.pdf.

→ RCPsych information on ADHD: http://www.rcpsych.ac.uk/healthadvice/parentsandyouthinfo/parentscarers/adhdhyperkineticdisorder.aspx.

20. **A** ★★★★ OHPsych 3rd edn → p.666

The technique of circular questioning (A), used in systemic and family therapy, aims at gathering and, at the same time, introducing information into the family system. The gathering of information aids in the formulation and validation of hypotheses regarding the family's dynamic structure. This form of questioning helps the therapist develop an understanding of how each member of the family experiences the current situation and how they respond to each other's responses. This builds a deeper understanding of the family relationships and dynamics present.

Direct questions (B) often result in short answers and do not lend themselves to exploring difficulties. Whilst it is likely that some direct questions will be asked, it will not be the dominant technique used in aiding the assessment of family dynamics.

Motivational questioning (C) is often used to assess motivation for change. It would not help assessment of the family dynamics.

Open questions (D) are questions used to get more information than just yes or no. This type of question is likely to be employed in the assessment but is not the most appropriate in assessing family dynamics.

Socratic questioning (E) has a systematic style, often challenging assumptions and underlying beliefs. It is primarily used in a therapeutic manner in CBT. It is not the most useful form of questioning in this context and is better used in individual therapy.

→ Perlmutter R (2004) *A Family Approach to Psychiatric Disorders*, Chapter 2, p.14. American Psychiatric Publishing, Arlington.

Extended Matching Questions

1. F ★

This man is presenting with intrusive obsessive thoughts about his family coming to harm which have been occurring over time. He has developed compulsions to try to counteract the thoughts. They are repetitive in nature, occurring every night, and causing him impairment, for which he has sought help.

2. I ★

This boy is presenting with symptoms of anxiety and distress specifically when separating from his primary caregiver. Most children experience some level of distress separating from parents. However, his distress is at levels beyond what is expected given that his mother still needs to remain in the classroom and he has not been able to attend a friend's house on his own yet.

3. A ★

This woman has experienced an acutely stressful event in the very recent past. It is very common for people who have experienced this to have symptoms of stress minutes to hours afterwards which can last up to a few days. These symptoms can include a feeling of numbness, confusion and disorientation, and autonomic symptoms of anxiety including tachycardia, flushing, and sweating. She is not presenting with PTSD, as there is a latency period of weeks to months for these symptoms to present.

4. C ★

Agoraphobia is a fairly well-defined cluster of phobias embracing fears of leaving home, entering shops, crowds and public places, or travelling alone on public transport. It also includes avoidance behaviours; for example, the woman now only shops online, suggesting she is avoiding going out to shop.

5. J ★

This man presents with a specific anxiety to social situations. He is reportedly managing to achieve well academically but avoiding social situations involving peers. His concerns about blushing and frequent micturition are common in people with this disorder. They fear scrutiny on a social level.

General feedback on 1–5: OHPsych 3rd edn → pp.54–5

→ Royal College of Psychiatry (RCPsych) information on obsessive compulsive disorder: http://www.rcpsych.ac.uk/mentalhealthinfo-forall/problems/obsessivecompulsivedisorder/obsessivecompulsive-disorder.aspx.

→ RCPsych information on coping with trauma: http://www.rcpsych.
ac.uk/expertadvice/problems/anxietyphobias/copingwithtrauma.aspx.

→ RCPsych information on shyness and social phobia: http://www.
rcpsych.ac.uk/expertadvice/problems/anxietyphobias/shynessandso-
cialphobia.aspx.

6. F ★

Perseveration is the persistent repetition of words or ideas. This may
involve repeatedly giving the same answer to different questions.

7. A ★

Circumstantiality is speech that is highly detailed and very delayed at
reaching its goal. The person may speak about many concepts related
to the point of the conversation before eventually returning to the point
and concluding the thought.

8. C ★

Echolalia is the echoing of one's or other people's speech that may only
be committed once or may be continuous in repetition. This may involve
only the last few words or last word of the examiner's sentences.

9. I ★

Thought insertion is a belief by a person that thoughts of other people
can be inserted into their own minds. It is an FRS.

10. D ★

Flight of ideas is a sequence of loose associations or extreme tangentiality where the speaker goes quickly from one seemingly unrelated idea
to another and that do not seem to repeat. Pressured speech is often
also present.

General feedback on 6–10: OHPsych 3rd edn → pp.62–5

→ Sims A (2002). Symptoms in the Mind: An Introduction to *Descriptive
Psychopathology*, 3rd edn, pp.149–88. Saunders, Philadelphia.

Chapter 3

Symptoms of psychiatric illness

Peter Sloan, Joy Bell, and Gil Myers

Few physical signs or investigative tools are available to psychiatrists to aid them in making their diagnosis. An ability to understand the patient's mental state is therefore of vital importance in categorizing and precisely communicating their mental disorder. The MSE is the psychiatrist's most used and useful resource. It elicits psychopathology in particular patterns, enabling diagnoses to be made.

Psychopathology can therefore be defined as the scientific study of abnormal experience, cognition, and behaviour (Sims, 2002) and was first described by Karl Jaspers in the early 1900s. More specifically, descriptive psychopathology is the *subjective* description of abnormal experience as related by patients and the *objective* observation of their behaviour.

It has facilitated the creation of diagnostic systems, for example ICD-10 and DSM-IV, grouping symptom clusters and classifying which signs and symptoms indicate a particular diagnosis.

In this chapter, you will be presented with a number of clinical scenarios, which will enable you to familiarize yourself with some of the important phenomenological terms used by clinicians to help classify experience and illness. We have attempted to incorporate signs encountered in all elements of the MSE and have used clinical examples from the main diagnostic groups.

Peter Sloan and Joy Bell

QUESTIONS

Single Best Answers

1. A 39-year-old man is assessed in a psychiatric outpatient clinic. He is referred because his partner is concerned that he is always worrying about their food being poisoned when they have meals outside their house. After a full assessment, a diagnosis of delusional disorder is made and treatment started. Which is the *single* most likely associated feature of this condition? ★

A Auditory hallucinations are a feature

B Delusions are bizarre in nature

C Delusions are circumscribed

D It is often co-morbid with schizophrenia

E There is a marked decline in social function

2. A 15-year-old adolescent is sent to the ED by her school nurse after she fainted at school. Her BMI is 17 kg/m². She says she feels cold and hungry. When asked, she says that her last period was three months ago. Her heart rate is 40 bpm and postural hypotension is elicited. Blood tests show hypokalaemia and hyponatraemia. Which is the *single* most likely diagnosis? ★

A Anorexia nervosa

B Bulimia nervosa

C Diabetes insipidus

D Paracetamol overdose

E Pregnancy

3. A 22-year-old man has a diagnosis of schizophrenia. He believes that members of the public are able to hear his thoughts being spoken aloud. Which is the *single* most appropriate description of this phenomenon? ★

A Thought block

B Thought broadcast

C Thought echo

D Thought insertion

E Thought withdrawal

4. An 81-year-old man with respiratory tract infection becomes acutely confused and agitated. Although this current confusion is thought to be due to delirium, he is also believed to have an undiagnosed dementia. Which *single* clinical finding most supports this additional diagnosis? ★

A Acute onset

B Diurnal variation in symptoms

C Fluctuating course

D Severe cognitive impairment

E Visual hallucinations

5. A 60–year-old woman is a surgical inpatient, recently diagnosed with metastatic breast carcinoma. She is found hanging in the bathroom of the surgical ward. She is rescued and later that day is assessed by the hospital liaison psychiatry team. Which is the *single* most significant indicator of suicidal intent in this case? ★

A At the time of the act she was being cared for 1:1 by nursing staff

B Her treatment was changed to palliative earlier that day

C History of deliberate self-harm (DSH) predating the diagnosis of malignancy

D She contacted her solicitor earlier that day to make a will

E The patient is a recent widow

6. A 25-year-old woman has low mood following the break-up of her relationship with her boyfriend of five years. She has read about her condition and believes she is having an 'adjustment reaction'. Her GP diagnoses her with a depressive episode. Which is the *single* feature that most supports the GP's diagnosis? ★

A The relationship ended yesterday

B Her speech is slow with long pauses before she answers

C She cries each time she looks at a photograph of her ex-boyfriend

D She has difficulty getting to sleep at night

E She is spending a lot of time with friends to take her mind off things

7. A 19-year-old man tells his GP that he is very concerned that a terrorist organization has bugged his house and is monitoring his every movement. He has no criminal record, no religious affiliations, and no concerns have previously been raised about his mental health. His GP described this in her referral as a primary, rather than a secondary, delusion. Which *single* feature, if present, makes this description more accurate? ★

A Appears suddenly as if 'out of the blue'

B Belief is understandable

C Belief precedes delusional atmosphere

D Can be traced in origin to the circumstances of his life

E Developed after auditory hallucinations

8. A 69-year-old man, who is a retired semi-professional rugby player, is depressed. He says he enjoys nothing in life, not even the Six Nations tournament, since his wife died eight months ago. Which is the *single* most appropriate description of this symptom? ★

A Anhedonia

B Masochism

C Nihilism

D Rumination

E Worthlessness

9. A 70-year-old man with vascular dementia is noted to have difficulty with his speech. After assessment it is apparent that he can speak fluently but cannot understand the words spoken to him. Which is the *single* most likely speech disorder he is displaying? ★

A Echolalia

B Expressive dysphasia

C Nominal aphasia

D Perseveration

E Receptive dysphasia

10. A 28-year-old man who has been on antipsychotic medication for schizophrenia for six months is restless and is constantly tapping his feet on the floor. Which is the *single* most likely motor symptom he is displaying? ★★

A Akathisia

B Chorea

C Mannerism

D Tardive dyskinesia

E Tics

11. A 68-year-old man is assessed by a liaison psychiatrist during a medical admission. He has a diagnosis of Alzheimer's dementia. Verbal perseveration is noted to be present. Which is the *single* most accurate statement regarding this symptom? ★★

A It always occurs in clouded consciousness

B It excludes a functional psychiatric illness

C It is categorized as a disorder of thought content

D It is observed in both motor and verbal modalities

E Perseveration can only be triggered by a question

12. A 42-year-old man has psychotic symptoms following the death of his sole surviving relative. A collateral history from a neighbour suggests that there has been 12 years of untreated psychosis. A diagnosis of catatonic schizophrenia is made. Which is the *single* most likely sign that will be observed? ★★

A Ataxic gait

B Circumstanciality

C Cogwheel rigidity

D Coprolalia

E Waxy flexibility

13. A 45-year-old man has been bereaved following the death of his wife three months ago. He feels sad and worthless and has been noted to be tearful, not enjoying his usual activities, and not sleeping well as he is waking early in the morning. He has a poor appetite and has lost weight. On several occasions he has heard the voice of his wife speaking to him. Which single symptom is the most indicative of an abnormal grief reaction? ★★

A Anhedonia

B Auditory hallucinations of the deceased

C Early morning wakening

D Feelings of worthlessness

E Weight loss

14. A 19-year-old student presents to her local ED with chest discomfort and shortness of breath. After extensive investigations, she is diagnosed with an acute anxiety attack. Which is the *single* most suggestive clinical indication for this diagnosis? ★★

A Arterial blood gas (ABG) shows a hypocapnic picture

B ECG shows second-degree heart block

C Her pain radiates to her left arm

D She has a history of congenital heart disease

E Symptoms settle following IV diamorphine

15. A 25-year-old man is preoccupied with the thought that his nose is too large and twisted to the left. Family and friends have tried to convince him that this is not the case. Which is the *single* most accurate statement regarding his situation? ★★

A Co-morbid depression is unlikely

B He will likely accept that the cause is psychological

C Surgery is the treatment of choice

D There is a high risk of self-mutilation

E This belief is delusional

16. A 50-year-old woman repeatedly goes to the local ED with a painful abdomen. She is investigated but no clear cause is found. After several presentations at different hospitals she is given a provisional diagnosis of Münchausen's syndrome. Which *single* feature would most strongly support this diagnosis? ★★

A Financial gain is consciously sought

B The information regarding her symptoms is mostly true

C The patient fabricates an illness in her child as well

D Her motivation is to receive attention and sympathy

E Her symptoms are implausible

17. A 24-year-old man, taking mood-stabilizing medication for BPAD, is found unconscious by his flatmates at 3 am covered in vomit. Earlier that day he told his flatmate he had split up with his boyfriend and felt 'awful'. He was seen to be a little drowsy in the evening but this wasn't taken seriously at the time. Which is the *single* most appropriate initial investigation to consider? ★★

A Computed tomography (CT) scan of the brain

B EEG

C Liver function test (LFT)

D UDS

E Valproate levels

18. A 70-year-old man is convinced that is wife is having an extra-marital affair. He has been following her secretly and checking her emails. A provisional diagnosis of morbid jealousy is made. Which *single* aspect of the assessment would make this diagnosis most likely? ★★★

A He copes with these concerns by drinking alcohol to excess

B He does not threaten violence to his wife's suspected sexual partner

C He has proof that his belief is based on true evidence

D He is reassured when his wife denies the accusations

E His wife states she has been unfaithful in the marriage

19. A 47-year-old women with benzodiazepine dependence requests a repeat prescription of lorazepam from her GP. She is suspected of having an acute benzodiazepine withdrawal. Which is the *single* most likely elicited clinical sign to suggest this diagnosis? ★★★

A Dilated pupils

B Drowsiness

C Fasciculations

D Piloerection

E Tachycardia

20. A 26-year-old woman is admitted to a neurology ward with lower limb paralysis. No medical cause is found. Her mental state is assessed and she is described as having 'la belle indifférence'. Which is the *single* most accurate statement regarding this diagnosis? ★★★★

A It describes the transfer of a delusional belief from one person to another

B It is a type of dissociation of affect

C It is an observation of a thought form

D It is common in patients with medically unexplained symptoms

E She is likely to be extremely distressed about her diagnosis

Extended Matching Questions

Alcohol side-effects

For each scenario below, choose the *single* most likely diagnosis from the list of options. Each option may be used once, more than once, or not at all. ★★

A Alcoholic blackouts

B Alcoholic cerebellar degeneration

C Alcoholic hallucinosis

D Central pontine myelinosis

E Delirium tremens

F Generalized cerebral atrophy

G Korsakoff's syndrome

H Post-acute-withdrawal syndrome

I Marchiafava–Bignami disease

J Wernicke's encephalopathy

1. A 56-year-old man is admitted to the medical ward. He is confused and has clouding of consciousness. He also has nystagmus, ocular palsy, ataxia, and peripheral neuropathy.

2. A 48-year-old man, who has been in police custody for the last 48 hours, is brought into the ED. Since his arrest he hasn't slept and has become more disorientated, labile in mood, and anxious. Now he has clouding of consciousness, tremor, and autonomic overarousal. He appears to be responding to visual hallucinations.

3. A 75-year-old widow is admitted to the medical ward for investigation of abnormal liver function. She has impaired STM, confabulation, and peripheral neuropathy.

4. A 60-year-old woman is brought to the ED by her daughter. She has auditory and visual hallucinations and says she can hear accusatory and threatening voices. She has no other physical symptoms. Her daughter tells you that she was a heavy drinker but has not had an alcoholic drink in the last 12–24 hours.

5. A 75-year-old homeless man is picked up by police because they suspect that he is drunk. He is brought to the ED and has impaired coordination and balance, tremor, truncal ataxia, impaired gait, and slowed and slurred speech.

Unusual syndromes

For each scenario below, choose the *single* most appropriate psychiatric syndrome from the list of options. Each option may be used once, more than once, or not at all. ★★★★

A Alice in Wonderland syndrome

B Briquet syndrome

C Capgras syndrome

D Cotard syndrome

E Ekbom syndrome

F Frégoli syndrome

G Ganser syndrome

H Kleine–Levin syndrome

I Münchausen syndrome

J Othello syndrome

6. A 26-year-old woman misidentifies a passenger on the bus as her mother in disguise, then later in the journey the accusation is made about a shop assistant, taxi driver, and passerby. This happens repeatedly throughout the day. She is very upset about her mother following her.

7. A 36-year-old prison inmate is asked 'What is the capital of Scotland?' and answers 'Paris'. When asked how many legs a dog has, he answers 'five'.

8. A 27-year-old woman describes seeing 'tiny little people' running about the garden and experiences an altered sense of velocity and perspective.

9. The family of a 15-year-old adolescent describes a pattern of difficult behaviour which involves periods of sustained overeating and daytime sleepiness where he will wake only to go to the toilet or to eat more. He is bedridden, uncommunicative, and unable to attend school.

10. A 25-year-old woman seeks treatment from her gynaecologist for multiple, recurring, unexplained symptoms. There is no evidence to suggest that these symptoms are being intentionally fabricated.

ANSWERS

Single Best Answers

1. C ★   OHPsych 3rd edn → pp.220–3

The answer is delusions are circumscribed (C). In delusional disorder, patients present with circumscribed, non-bizarre delusions, in the absence of thought disorder or significant blunting of affect. This means that the delusions do not prevent general logical reasoning outside the scope of the delusion, and there is usually no overt disturbance of behaviour. If there is any disturbed behaviour it is directly related to the delusional belief. A number of subtypes exist including erotomania type, grandiose type, and jealousy type.

For a diagnosis to be made, auditory and visual hallucinations cannot be prominent (A), although olfactory or tactile hallucinations related to the content of the delusion may be present.

In delusional disorders the delusions are fixed false beliefs focused around scenarios which could possibly occur in real life; for example, a house being watched for a burglary. It is usually the persistent nature of the belief and its unshakable value that starts to alert other people that there is a problem. Thus (B) is not a correct answer.

Neither is (D). Delusional disorder is not diagnosed if there is already a diagnosis of schizophrenia or an affective disorder. Also, substance misuse must first be ruled out. It usually presents in middle to late adult life, and is more common in women than men. In particular, recent immigrants are at higher risk.

In chronic delusional disorders there does not need to be social isolation or a decline in social function (E). Often people will keep their 'odd' beliefs hidden or only reveal them to certain, trusted people. As they are not too bizarre they can be ignored or minimized by others.

2. A ★   OHPsych 3rd edn → pp. 75–6, 399–401

The answer is anorexia nervosa (A). Physical consequences of anorexia nervosa include hypotension, bradycardia, hypokalaemia, and hyponatraemia (amongst a range of multisystem complications). Cardiac complications are the most common cause of death in this disorder with a 10% mortality rate. BMI is diagnostically under 17.5 kg/m^2.

Body weight is more likely to be normal in bulimia nervosa (B), though metabolic disturbances due to purging may also result in hypokalaemia and hyponatraemia.

Classic symptoms of diabetes insipidus (C) are of excessive thirst and excessive urine production.

As paracetamol is not sedative, drowsiness or loss of consciousness is not seen after overdose (D). Be aware that some painkiller preparations contain paracetamol and codeine; here sedation may be seen in overdose due to the effects of the codeine. Coma and death may be seen as late complications of untreated paracetamol overdose due to fulminant hepatic failure.

Pregnancy (E) may cause nausea and feeling faint, but would not normally result in the metabolic disturbances in this scenario. Period irregularity or amenorrhea are commonly seen in anorexia where hormone levels are affected by inadequate nutrition.

3. B ★   OHPsych 3rd edn → pp.62–4

Thought broadcast (B) is the belief that others are able to access an individual's thoughts or that they are being spoken aloud and therefore others can hear them. It is an FRS of schizophrenia.

Thought block (A) is the sudden arrest of the train of thought. True thought block is suggestive of schizophrenia but it is not an FRS—for this to be an FRS the thought must have been subjectively (i.e. explained by the patient as being) withdrawn.

Thought echo (C) is an auditory hallucination and an FRS of schizophrenia. The patient describes hearing their own thoughts spoken aloud after the thought has occurred.

Thought insertion (D) is the belief that a foreign thought is being inserted into the mind. This thought is inserted from outside the head, as opposed to a thought in OCD where the origin is the patient's own thoughts, however unwelcome. This is a delusional belief most commonly associated with schizophrenia.

Thought withdrawal (E) is the belief that thoughts are being withdrawn from the mind by an outside influence. When the thought is described as being withdrawn (rather than just disappearing) it is considered an FRS of schizophrenia. Therefore it is important to clarify with the patient by direct questioning what they believe is happening.

→ Casey P, Kelly B (2007). *Fish's Clinical Psychopathology*, 3rd edn, p.38. RCPsych Publications, London.

4. D ★   OHPsych 3rd edn → pp.132–3, 146, 790–3

Severe cognitive impairment (D) is more likely with dementia. Though a severe episode of delirium can also cause this, it is usually less severe, and the fluctuating course of delirium means it is unlikely to persist.

Acute onset does not support this diagnosis (A). Both delirium and dementia are heterogeneous conditions that can cause a wide range of symptoms and signs. No individual finding is pathognomic of one or the other, and must be interpreted in the context of the whole clinical picture. Furthermore, in older people, a delirium can arise on top of an underlying dementia (which in turn makes delirium more likely to occur) that may or may not have been previously diagnosed. Most dementias present insidiously over a prolonged period of time. Rarer dementias such as Creutzfeldt–Jakob could potentially present more acutely, but this would be a rare finding.

Delirium classically presents with diurnal variation in symptoms (B), which can make its identification difficult. However, patients with Alzheimer's disease also experience 'sun-downing', where there is a worsening of symptoms in the evening time.

Classically, the time course of delirium is one of fluctuations (C), while dementias are more progressive. However, Lewy body dementia presents with a fluctuating time course and the step-wise progression of vascular dementias can be difficult to distinguish from this clinically.

Visual hallucinations (E) can be found in both conditions, though in dementia it would be more likely in advanced stages.

5. D ★   OHPsych 3rd edn → pp.52, 987

Contacting her solicitor earlier that day to make a will (D) is the most significant indicator of suicidal intent. In this case, the final act of making a will is most indicative of suicidal intent. It is suggestive of forward planning, a wish to end her life, and some degree of logical thinking. All of these are high-risk acts.

At the time of the act she was being cared for 1:1 by nursing staff (A) and this is actually protective, as self-harm in the presence of a nurse, or any carer, may indicate a desire to be intercepted.

Without knowing more about her treatment change and her reaction to this it is hard to judge the implication of a change to palliative treatment earlier that day (B). In these kinds of palliative decisions, the aim is to act in accordance with the patient's wishes and to counsel them about the decision.

A history of self-harm, although increasing her risk of completed suicide, is not necessarily linked to intent at this particular point (C).

Even if the patient is a recent widow (E), this does not necessarily mean that she is upset to be so, or that it has impacted on her mood. To a lesser extent, the prognosis of her illness and her demographic, in the context of a comprehensive risk assessment, may also contribute to changes in her affect, but they need to be explored. It is important to deal in facts and evidence rather than judgements.

6. B ★   OHPsych 3rd edn → pp.386–7

Slow speech with long pauses before answering (B) supports the diagnosis. Psychomotor retardation is a feature of depressive illness which is not normally seen in other causes of low mood, such as situational crisis. Depression would also typically be associated with anhedonia (loss of interest), decreased appetite and weight loss, diurnal mood variation, and poor concentration, and often the patient self-isolates. Delay in speech production and decreased volume and speed of speech are indicative.

If the relationship ended yesterday this does not support the diagnosis (A). A depressive episode is diagnosed when five or more depressive symptoms have been present for longer than two weeks, irrespective of the close temporal relationship between an identifiable stressor and symptoms. An adjustment disorder is diagnosed within one month of the stressor.

Crying each time she looks at a photograph of her ex-boyfriend (C) is not pathognomonic for depression, or for an adjustment disorder. It is common after many break-ups, no matter how serious they were.

Difficulty in getting to sleep at night (D) is present in a number of situations and not indicative of any single diagnosis—or even of a mental illness.

If she were depressed then it would be more likely that she has anhedonia and would be spending time with friends (E). She would be unlikely to find that she could 'take her mind off things'.

→ http://bjp.rcpsych.org/content/179/6/479.full

→ Casey P (2001). Adjustment disorders. *British Journal of Psychiatry*, **179**, 479–81.

→ Sims A (2002). *Symptoms in the Mind: An Introduction to Descriptive Psychopathology*, 4th edn, pp.158–9. Saunders, Philadelphia.

7. A ★   OHPsych 3rd edn → pp. 90–1

Primary delusions by definition characteristically appear 'out of the blue' (A). Delusional mood, delusional memory, autochthonous delusions, and delusional perception are all types of primary delusion.

Primary delusions were described by Jaspers as being 'ultimately un-understandable' as they do not arise from a pre-existing concept (B). There is no reason to disbelieve a patient's claims, but common sense should be used and evidence sought to confirm or deny these claims.

A delusional atmosphere is synonymous with delusion mood. This is a form of primary delusion which is recalled after the delusional belief is perceived, not preceding it (C). For example, the patient feels on edge, anxious, and hyperaware, then has a realization (the delusional belief) which makes his anxiety appear justified.

Andrew Sims in his book *Symptoms in the Mind* explains that primary delusions are not amenable to logic and the absurdity or erroneousness of their content is manifest to other people. There is no evidence here that there is any origin to these beliefs in this patient's life (D).

Auditory hallucinations are part of FRS (of schizophrenia) but separate from delusions. They can occur independently and are not time dependent on delusional beliefs (E).

→ Sims A (2002). *Symptoms in the Mind: An Introduction to Descriptive Psychopathology*, 4th edn, pp.124–31. Saunders, Philadelphia.

8. A ★   OHPsych 3rd edn → pp.50–1, 86

Anhedonia (A) is an inability to experience pleasure, characteristically a symptom of depression. People suffering with depression tend to lose interest in things they once found enjoyable. Activities are no longer enjoyable and there is often a loss of interest in or desire for sex. In this case, the patient says that he enjoys nothing, not even something we assume he will relish. Once depression is resolved, the enjoyment of activities is expected to return and therefore it is important to encourage patients not to abandon their social contacts, sports equipment, etc., even if they are not currently using them.

Masochism (B) is the act of gaining gratification from pain or degradation inflicted on oneself. It can be due to one's own actions or the actions of others. There is no evidence that this man shows any enjoyment at preventing himself from watching the rugby. Often masochism is paired with sadism where the other person enjoys the act of inflicting pain. There is no established link between depression and masochism (or sadism)—although Freud believed that both were integral to psychoanalysis and sexual intercourse.

Nihilism (C) is a rejection of traditional beliefs which argues that life is without objective meaning or value. In psychiatry, most often in schizophrenia, patients have a nihilistic delusion which is the (false) belief that they have died and therefore no longer exist. Because it is a delusional belief it lacks the logical counter-argument which asks how it is possible for the person to be answering questions if they are dead.

Rumination (D) is the repetitive, frequent focus on past negative events or feelings. Often ruminations are part of the depressive picture and can contribute to the length of the depressive episode. They are much like a compulsion in that they are not easy to stop, and cause distress. Ruminations tend to be focused on past events, as opposed to anxieties which are more concerned with potential problems in the future.

Depressed people can view themselves as worthless (E). Thoughts of this kind are biased in a negative manner, focusing on mistakes, failing, and poor performance in the past in an unhealthy and unrealistic way. Often they will consider that they had more control, even choice, over these events and should have been able to prevent them. While this man may have this, it is not the symptom described.

9. E ★ OHPsych 3rd edn → pp.95, 103

The answer is receptive dysphasia (E). This describes the loss of comprehension of the meaning of words and of the significance of grammar. Speech is fluent.

Echolalia (A) is the repetition of words or phrases that are spoken to a patient. There is normally no understanding of their meaning. It occurs in catatonic schizophrenia and dementia.

Expressive dysphasia (B) is a motor speech disturbance where there is difficulty selecting words, constructing sentences, and expressing them. Understanding is often preserved.

In nominal aphasia (C) the patient is unable to produce the names of objects at will.

Perseveration (D) occurs with clouded consciousness. It describes the phenomenon where a response that was appropriate to a first stimulus (or question) is given inappropriately to subsequent questions.

→ Sims A (2002). *Symptoms in the Mind: An Introduction to Descriptive Psychopathology*, 4th edn, pp.177–82. Saunders, Philadelphia.

10. **A** ★★ OHPsych 3rd edn → pp.86–8, 99, 104–5

The answer is akathisia (A). This is a subjective sense of an uncomfortable desire to move—described by some as an 'inner restlessness'. It is relieved by repeated movement of the affected part (usually the legs). While it can be resisted, unlike tardive dyskinesia, this require a large amount of effort and concentration. It is a common side-effect of antipsychotic treatment and is treated by withdrawing or decreasing the dose, which normally causes a reduction in the symptoms.

Chorea (B) is the sudden and involuntary movement of several muscles in the body with a resultant dance-like movement of the body. It occurs in the genetic condition Huntington's chorea.

Mannerisms (C) are abnormal and sometimes bizarre actions which are produced in a goal-directed fashion. This can include abnormal walking and gestures.

Tardive dyskinesia (D) is a movement disorder that is associated with long-term use of antipsychotic medication. There are continuous involuntary movements of the tongue and lower face.

A tic (E) is a sudden twitch of a single muscle or muscle group. It can occur in various conditions, including Gilles de la Tourette's syndrome where tics can be motor or verbal.

11. **D** ★★ OHPsych 3rd edn → p.101

Verbal perseveration is observed in both motor and verbal modalities (D). Perseveration is the persistent repetition of the same verbal or motor response to varied stimuli with continuance of activity after cessation of the causative stimulus.

Verbal perseveration occurs in clouded consciousness with organic states, but can occur in clear conscious states such as schizophrenia (A).

It excludes a functional psychiatric illness (B) is not the right answer. Verbal perseveration can occur in schizophrenia and organic states.

Verbal perseveration is not categorized as a disorder of thought content or motor speech (C).

Verbal perseveration may be produced spontaneously or may be set off by a question (E).

→ Casey P, Kelly B (2007). *Fish's Clinical Psychopathology*, 3rd edn, p.98. RCPsych Publications, London.

→ Sims A (2002). *Symptoms in the Mind: An Introduction to Descriptive Psychopathology*, 3rd edn, pp.70-1. Saunders, Philadelphia.

12. **E** ★★ OHPsych 3rd edn → p.167

The answer is waxy flexibility (E). This is the plastic resistance encountered on moulding the limbs of a patient with catatonia. When passive movement stops the final posture is preserved and can include uncomfortable positions.

Ataxic gait (A) is seen in cerebellar lesions.

Circumstanciality (B) is the inclusion of unnecessary and trivial detail in conversation.

Cogwheel rigidity (C) is a feature of parkinsonism.

Coprolalia (D) is a forced vocalization which often takes the form of obscene words or phrases. It is observed in Gilles de la Tourette's syndrome.

→ Casey P, Kelly B (2007). *Fish's Clinical Psychopathology*, 3rd edn, p.99. RCPsych Publications, London.

→ Sims A (2002). *Symptoms in the Mind: An Introduction to Descriptive Psychopathology*, 3rd edn,p p.383–4. Saunders, Philadelphia.

13. D ★★   OHPsych 3rd edn → p.388–9

The symptom most indicative of this condition is a feeling of worthlessness (D). It is more likely to occur in an abnormal grief reaction and is indicative of depression. A typical grief reaction may last around six months, but can be up to one year. In "normal" grief people may experience disbelief, shock, anger, low mood, tearfulness, irritability, anhedonia, early morning wakening, loss of appetite, weight and libido. Over time these symptoms diminish in intensity with gradual acceptance. A third of bereaved people would meet diagnostic criteria for a depressive episode at some point. Abnormal grief is characterized by intense, prolonged or delayed symptoms. There may be feelings of worthlessness, excessive guilt, suicidal ideation, functional impairment, psychomotor retardation, or persistent hallucinations which require active treatment rather than supportive care.

Anhedonia (A) is the loss of enjoyment in previously pleasurable activities. It often appears in normal bereavement, maybe in part due to the loss of the a partner in shared activities or feelings of guilt at enjoying an activity without the deceased.

Auditory hallucinations (B) of the dead person can occur in normal bereavement. They are often more common early on in the bereavement process (i.e. soon after death) and are more prevalent in cultures where the dead speaking is considered more acceptable.

Early morning waking (C) is more often a symptom of depression, it can occur in normal bereavement. Often it is due to lifestyle changes, for example sleeping in an empty double bed.

Weight loss (E) can occur in normal bereavement due to a change in lifestyle, for example this patient may not know how to cook food as it was always his wife's role in the household. It can also be associated with depression as part of a self-neglecting presentation.

14. A ★★   OHPsych 3rd edn → pp.54–5, 781

ABG showing a hypocapnic picture is the most suggestive clinical indication for the diagnosis (A). Hyperventilation during a panic attack 'blows off' carbon dioxide, leading to reduced serum levels on ABG sampling.

ECG shows that second-degree heart block is not suggestive as heart block is not a feature of anxiety. ECG may show sinus tachycardia.

Radiation of pain to the left arm (C) is indicative of acute coronary syndrome.

Anxiety disorder is not associated with congenital heart disease (D).

Diamorphine (E) may have an anxiolytic effect, but answer (A) is more indicative of acute anxiety.

→ NICE Clinical Guideline 113—Anxiety: http://guidance.nice.org.uk/CG113.

15. D ★★   OHPsych 3rd edn → p.810

There have been cases where patients buy surgical kits and perform 'self-surgery' (D). This is difficult to prevent as it is a condition associated with social isolation and lack of help-seeking behaviour.

'Co-morbid depression is unlikely' is not the most accurate statement (A). Often patients with this body dysmorphic disorder (BDD) describe depressed mood, anxiety, and social isolation. It is difficult to pull apart which came first as it is often a culmination of factors. It is known to have precipitating factors in bullying, eating disorders, and social phobia.

The statement 'He will likely accept that the cause is psychological' (B) is not most accurate. Often these patients are very frustrated by having to see psychiatry doctors, as they want to have surgery. Psychiatric investigation scales used for BDD are the Body Dysmorphic Disorder Examination Sheet and the Yale–Brown Obsessive Compulsive Scale modified for BDD. In many ways, BDD is similar to OCD in its obsessional quality and compulsive behaviours. In BDD the compulsions may be mental compulsions, for example the patient thinking about how they look as a 'mental mirror', rather than physical rituals.

Surgical intervention is unhelpful as the belief remains (C). Most patients with BDD will have sought an assessment or treatment from a cosmetic surgeon. Usually surgery will result in a reduction in symptoms for a time before the anxieties return in the same manner, or move to a different body area. This can mean multiple surgeries and huge sums of money spent. Research has been conducted on BDD by assessing all patients waiting in plastic surgery waiting rooms. CBT is the treatment of choice, with the use of selective serotonin reuptake inhibitors (SSRIs) if the diagnosis is entrenched. The evidence is that the dose of antidepressant needed to treat BDD is higher than that for depression or OCD.

This belief is not delusional (E) but is an overvalued idea and the patient normally can gain a degree of insight. For a diagnosis of BDD to be reached, the object of concern must be within the normal range and not be considered a disfigurement.

→ Sims A (2002). *Symptoms in the Mind: An Introduction to Descriptive Psychopathology*, 4th edn, pp.268–70. Saunders, Philadelphia.

→ Veale D (2010). *Body Dysmorphic Disorder*. http://www.veale.co.uk/resources-support/public-information/body-dysmorphic-disorder.

16. D ★★   OHPsych 3rd edn → pp.814–15

Motivation to receive attention and sympathy (D) most strongly supports this diagnosis. Fabricated or induced illness comprises intentional production or feigning of medical symptoms with repeated hospital attendances. The motivation for the behaviour is to assume the sick role.

Financial gain is consciously sought (A) is the wrong answer. In fabricated or induced illness, previously called Münchausen syndrome, external incentives for the behaviour (such as economic gain, avoiding legal responsibility, or improving physical wellbeing) are absent. If they are present then a diagnosis of malingering is more appropriate.

The information regarding her symptoms is mostly true (B) is also incorrect. As with any fabricated story, there are often many elements that are true partly as it makes it easier to remember and maintain a story. There are some case studies to suggest that this is a learnt behaviour from a previous illness where the care received 'legitimately' is idealized and sought after again.

Fabricated or induced illness by carers, or, as it also known, medical child abuse or Münchausen's by proxy, is a relatively rare form of child abuse which involves an adult, usually the mother or carer, in the fabrication of illnesses in a child or person under their care (C). There is debate if there is also a secondary gain for the perpetrator as they have 'got one over' on medical professionals. This is a notoriously difficult form of abuse to confirm—most recently it has been seen in veterinary surgeries with people fabricating illnesses in their animals to receive sympathy from vets.

Often initial symptoms are plausible and, with repeated presentations, some patients learn which are the 'red flag' symptoms to mention in order to raise anxiety and ensure admission. Therefore (E) is not the correct answer. As the admission progresses, however, symptoms can become extremely improbable, including new important but forgotten parts of the past medical history. With access to the internet it is becoming increasingly easy to fake complicated illnesses.

→ Sims A (2002). *Symptoms in the Mind: An Introduction to Descriptive Psychopathology*, 4th edn, pp.265–7. Saunders, Philadelphia.

17. E ★★   OHPsych 3rd edn → pp.576, 928

Valproate (E) is widely used as a mood stabilizer in BPAD. Although most cases of valproate overdose are benign, serious toxicity, including death, may occur after acute ingestion. Gastrointestinal (GI) upset with nausea and vomiting is the most common presentation, closely followed by central nervous system (CNS) symptoms of decreased level of consciousness and confusion. If an enteric coated formulation of valproate has been ingested then it may form concretions in the GI tract, which means absorption may be delayed and prolonged. Assessing levels is essential in determining treatment.

If the patient is unconscious and unresponsive then a UDS (D) is more difficult to obtain. It would be faster and more efficient to treat the likely causative agents than to waste time searching for unlikely ones.

Imaging of this kind is more helpful in traumatic brain injury. If, in this instance, there was such an injury, the fact that he has a decreased Glasgow Comma Scale (GCS) score and vomiting would mean that a CT scan should be requested immediately. However, without a brain injury, it's a second-line investigation (A).

An EEG (B) would not be a first-line investigation in this instance. It is time consuming and unlikely to change treatment choices.

LFTs (C) are not the most appropriate initial investigation. Although hepatotoxicity may occasionally occur with overdose, this is more of a chronic effect seen in therapeutic doses and occurs most commonly in the first few months of treatment. It is not something that should be treated at this emergency stage.

18. A ★★★ OHPsych 3rd edn → pp.100, 569

Coping with these concerns by drinking alcohol to excess (A) is the single aspect of the assessment that would make this diagnosis most likely. Morbid jealousy is a delusional disorder most common in males associated with alcohol dependence, impotence, and different forms of dementia. Morbid jealousy is also known as 'Othello syndrome' from the character in Shakespeare's play *Othello* who murders his wife as a result of a false belief that she has been unfaithful.

Patients with morbid jealousy will often make threats against their partner or their partner's 'lover' and there have been cases where one or both have been killed. Morbid jealousy is one of the commonest motivations for homicide, and in fact geographical separation of the couple may at times be necessary as it can be very difficult to treat with medication. It would be very unlikely that this man would not have threatened his wife or her 'partner' in the context of this jealous belief (B).

Even if the patient is reassured that they are wrong, they will not be able to maintain this belief and prevent their obsessional thoughts, much in the same way that a patient with OCD regarding germs may understand that they 'can't' catch HIV from a toilet seat will still finds it impossible not to worry about the possibility that doctors may be wrong (C).

If he is reassured when his wife denies the accusations (D) the belief is based on 'delusional evidence', which may be a relatively meaningless event or object with a delusional meaning attached. An example would be if her husband found a phone number in her phone that was unknown to him he may believe this means her new partner has been contacting her. Therefore any denial will be ignored because this is not a logical, or understandable, belief.

In morbid jealousy there is no proof that infidelity, or lack thereof, has any bearing on the diagnosis. A patient can still meet the criteria for morbid jealousy even if there is an affair and therefore there is something to be jealous of (E).

→ Casey P, Kelly B (2007). *Fish's Clinical Psychopathology*, 3rd edn, p.125. RCPsych Publications, London.

→ Sims A (2002). *Symptoms in the Mind: An Introduction to Descriptive Psychopathology*, 4th edn, pp.136-7. Saunders, Philadelphia.

19. A ★★★   OHPsych 3rd edn → pp.60, 582

Dilated pupils (A) along with tachycardia, hyperreflexia, and anxiety are signs of benzodiazepine withdrawal. Dilated pupils can also be seen in opiate withdrawal.

Drowsiness (B) is not commonly seen in benzodiazepine withdrawal, whereas restlessness is common. Drowsiness alongside headache, irritability, inability to concentrate, and joint pain are signs of caffeine withdrawal. These may appear within a day of discontinuation, peaking at around 48 hours, and lasting up to nine days. Caffeine withdrawal has now been categorized as a mental illness in DSM-V.

Fasciculations (C) are seen more commonly within alcohol withdrawal syndrome. In 'uncomplicated alcohol withdrawal syndrome' there can also be insomnia, headache, diaphoresis, nausea, and vomiting. The presence of any psychotic symptoms, confusion, or seizures suggests a 'complicated alcohol withdrawal syndrome'.

The classic triad for opioid withdrawal is piloerection (D), rhinorrhea, and lacrimation. While opioid withdrawal is uncomfortable it is not life-threatening, in contrast with alcohol and benzodiazepine withdrawal which are potentially life-threatening.

Tachycardia (E) is seen in benzodiazepine withdrawal but also in withdrawal from most illicit drugs (and many drug intoxications), as well as anxiety, illness, and other organic causes. This is too common a symptom to act as a definitive indicator of a specific drug withdrawal.

→ Sadock BJ, Sadock VA (2010). *Kaplan and Saddock's Pocket Handbook of Clinical Psychiatry*, 5th revised edn, p.397-8. Lippincott Williams and Wilkins, Philadelphia.

→ Taylor, D, Paton C, Kapur S (2012). *The Maudsley Prescribing Guidelines in Psychiatry*, 11th edn, p.306-309. Wiley, Chichester.

20. B ★★★★   OHPsych 3rd edn → p.88

La belle indifférence is a type of dissociation of affect (B) which is rare nowadays but which is well reported in psychiatric literature. It describes the apparent lack of distress caused by disabling symptoms of a conversion disorder. Usually the physical symptoms relieve anxiety and result in secondary gains in the form of sympathy and attention given by healthcare professionals and others.

Although the symptoms or are not intentionally fabricated they are not delusional. They also remain with the person expressing the belief rather than being transferred to another person (A). The diagnosis referred to in this description is 'Folie à deux' or shared psychosis.

There is no evidence that this is an observation of thought form (C), which are more around disordered thinking and speech such as derailment, tangentially, and thought withdrawal.

In patients with medically unexplained symptoms (D) there is often acute distress regarding these unexplained symptoms and a desire to solve them.

For 'la belle indifférence' to be diagnosed there must be a lack of distress which accompanies the physical symptoms (E).

→ Casey P, Kelly B (2007). *Fish's Clinical Psychopathology*, 3rd edn, p.68. RCPsych Publications, London.

→ Stone J, Smyth R, Carson A, Sharpe M (2006). La belle indifférence in conversion symptoms and hysteria. *British Journal of Psychiatry*, 188, 204–9.

Extended Matching Questions

1. J ★★

Wernicke's classic 'triad' is confusion, opthalmoplegia, and ataxia, although all three in combination are only seen in about 10% of cases. Amongst features of alcohol withdrawal, nystagmus and ocular palsies are unique to Wernicke's encephalopathy. Treatment is with parenteral thiamine.

2. E ★★

The giveaway sign of delirium tremens is autonomic overarousal. It can be distinguished from alcoholic hallucinosis on the basis of delayed onset, physical symptoms in addition to hallucinations, and possible mortality.

3. G ★★

Confabulation is a pathognomonic of Korsakoff's syndrome (also termed Korsakoff's psychosis, although it is not a psychotic disorder). Korsakoff's is considered an alcohol-related dementia but is also found in other chronic thiamine deficiency states. Wernicke–Korsakoff's syndrome is now considered to be a unitary disorder comprising acute Wernicke's encephalopathy, which proceeds in a proportion of cases to Korsakoff's syndrome. Increased vulnerability is associated with genetic susceptibility in association with poor diet.

4. C ★★

Alcoholic hallucinosis is distinct from delirium tremens in that it has a more rapid onset after cessation of drinking, involves a limited set of hallucinations and no other physical symptoms, and rarely results in death. Post-acute-withdrawal syndrome tends to occur a few weeks after stopping, with fewer physical symptoms but more emotional and psychological withdrawal symptoms.

5. B ★★

The giveaway is that all symptoms are clearly associated with cerebellar dysfunction, without the rest of Wernicke's triad.

General feedback on 1–5: OHPsych 3rd edn → pp.546–7, 558–9, 566–9

6. F ★★★★

In Frégoli syndrome the patient believes that an individual, most often unknown to them, is actually someone they know 'in disguise'. Usually the individual is thought to be pursuing or persecuting the patient in some way. The condition is named after the Italian actor Leopoldo Frégoli, who was renowned for his ability to make quick changes of appearance during his stage act.

7. G ★★★★

Ganser syndrome is characterized by the production of 'approximate answers'. The patient gives repeated wrong answers to simple questions, which are none the less almost correct. It is usually present with three other symptoms, called Ganser symptoms: psychogenic physical symptoms, visual pseudohallucinations, and amnesia for the period of the illness. It has been observed in prisoners awaiting trial, but is thought to occur more widely where there is reaction to extreme stress.

8. A ★★★★

Alice in Wonderland syndrome (sometimes known as Todd's syndrome) is a neurological disorder in which the patient's perceptions of body image, space, and time are distorted. Patients may experience micropsia, macropsia, or size distortions in other sensory modalities. Hallucinations in which things, people, or animals seem smaller than they would be in real life are called Lilliputian hallucination and have also been reported in this syndrome.

9. H ★★★★

Kleine–Levin syndrome is a rare disorder characterized by periodic somnolence and intense hunger. It occurs almost exclusively in male adolescents. It usually follows a course of decreasing frequency of attacks but may persist for many years before complete cessation.

10. B ★★★★

Briquet syndrome, or somatization disorder, is a chronic disorder characterized by multiple medically unexplained symptoms. For a diagnosis, multiple and variable physical symptoms must persist for two years. Patients refuse to accept advice or reassurance from medical experts that there is no physical explanation. If symptoms were thought to be intentionally fabricated this could indicate a diagnosis of 'fabricated or induced illness'.

General feedback on 6–10: OHPsych 3rd edn → pp.94–6, 434, 802–3, 911; ICD-10 → p.163

Community psychiatry

Andrew Watson and Gil Myers

An inpatient admission to a psychiatry ward has a high cost both economically and psychologically. While it is necessary at times to treat someone in hospital, the majority of the work in maintaining good mental health is done while the patient is living their usual life with its highs, lows, and challenges. Community psychiatry aims to manage people with mental illness in their own environment. There are many benefits to this, including promoting a sense of normality, allowing for continued support from family and friends, and helping to bridge the change between illness and recovery. Because of this, community psychiatry covers almost everything in psychiatry and is as much a speciality of exclusion as a specific group: no under 18s (child and adolescent), over 65s (psychiatry of old age), addictions (substance misuse), or the law (forensic psychiatry). But a community psychiatrist can't be too exclusive because local differences, based on what other dedicated services are available, and sub-threshold presentations mean that a good working knowledge of most conditions is essential. In many ways, community psychiatrists are the GPs of the speciality.

The only way to manage such a large and varied workload is to make good use of the multidisciplinary team (MDT): community psychiatric nurses (CPNs), occupational therapists (OTs), speech and language therapists (SALTs)—the list of acronyms is endless but essential. A good community psychiatrist has a team they can rely on to help keep a watchful eye over their clinical population; managing their day-to-day care and anticipating problems before a relapse develops. The balance between giving space for recovery and monitoring to ensure efficient treatment is hard to achieve but gratifying when it occurs.

Part of the skill set of a good community psychiatrist is an understanding of the research statistics: prevalence of disorders, treatment rates, and prognosis. These allow for faster diagnosis and evidence-based treatments to speed up recuperation. The minutiae of these facts aren't needed, but a broad understanding helps shape assessment and management.

Gil Myers

QUESTIONS

Single Best Answers

1. A 23-year-old man has never had a girlfriend. He has longstanding difficulties with social communication, although his language developmental milestones were normal and he passed two A-levels. He collects vintage comic books and spends the majority of his free time organizing this collection. He has been brought for assessment by his mother who is concerned, even though the man himself is not worried. Which is the *single* most likely diagnosis? ★

A Asperger's syndrome

B Autism

C Mild learning disability

D Paranoid PD

E Schizotypal disorder

2. A 23-year-old man has intense episodes of difficulty breathing and sweating, and feels his heart pounding. These last about 15 minutes. A recent one happened when he was sitting watching TV and another whilst he was using a photocopier at work. Which is the *single* most likely diagnosis? ★

A Agoraphobia

B Depression

C OCD

D Panic disorder

E Social phobia

3. A 41-year-old woman has lethargy, is very cold all the time, and feels low in her mood. Using the internet, she has diagnosed herself as having a moderate depressive illness. Which is the *single* most likely differential diagnosis? ★

A Glioma

B Hypercalcaemia

C Hypothyroidism

D Sleep apnoea

E Steroid use

4. A 21-year-old woman has concerns about her weight. She cannot stand the thought of being fat. At least four times a week she eats large quantities of crisps and chocolate and during these periods feels like she is losing control. Afterwards she runs a minimum of 10 km to 'burn off the calories'. Her BMI is 19 kg/m². Which is the *single* most likely diagnosis? ★

A Anorexia nervosa

B Binge-eating disorder

C Bulimia nervosa

D Delusional disorder

E Olympic training

5. A substantial proportion of people with mental health problems do not attend their doctor for assistance. Household surveys allow estimates of the prevalence in the whole community. Which *single* anxiety disorder is most likely to be found as the highest in such surveys? ★

A Agoraphobia

B Generalized anxiety disorder

C OCD

D Panic disorder

E Social phobia

6. A 26-year-old woman with anorexia nervosa is told that if she does not engage with her management plan she may require inpatient care in the future. Which is the *single* most likely indicator that this is necessary? ★

A Body temperature 35.5°C

B Difficult family dynamics

C Need to start antidepressants

D Starting a pro-ana blog

E Use of diet pills

7. A 41-year-old man reports seeing an explosion of colourful fireworks whenever he hears a car sounding its horn. He has used LSD for a number of years although says that this can happen when he isn't under the influence of the drug. Which is the *single* most appropriate description of his hallucination? ★

A Command hallucination

B Elementary hallucination

C Extracampine hallucination

D Gedankenlautwerden

E Reflex hallucination

8. A 22-year-old man has been performing poorly at his job for four months, around the time he started working at a new firm in a new town. He is unable to focus because he says he needs to get 'everything in order' and so he is generally slow in completing tasks. He has started to avoid after-work social events because he is afraid of contracting infections. He knows that having these thoughts are 'odd' but he can't seem to stop the worries they create. Other colleagues have noticed a change in his behaviour and started to gossip about him. Which is the *single* most likely diagnosis? ★

A Adjustment disorder

B Early-onset psychosis

C OCD

D Panic disorder

E PTSD

9. A 23-year-old is experiencing his first episode of psychosis. At times he is disorganized and distressed, but there is no history of any risk to himself or others. He lives at home, has a supportive family, and is keen to engage with services. Which *single* service is most appropriate for his care? ★

A Early intervention service

B General hospital inpatient care

C Primary care

D Psychiatric inpatient care

E Rehabilitation service

10. A 23-year-old man has had ten panic attacks in the last month. These can happen at any time. He is now very concerned about having another one. Which is the *single* most effective intervention to offer him? ★

A Amitriptyline 75 mg OD

B CBT

C Diazepam 5 mg OD

D Flooding

E Self-help book

11. A 29-year-old woman has relapsing BPAD. She has returned from a three-year stay in China where she did not take any medication. However, she is now planning to become pregnant and would like to know which prophylactic medication is recommended. Which is the *single* most appropriate initial medication to suggest? ★

A Carbamazepine

B Lithium

C Olanzapine

D Paroxetine

E Sodium valproate

12. A 35-year-old man registers with a GP surgery as a temporary patient. He says he is on a methadone programme in a different city and takes methadone 40 mg OD. As he is currently visiting his sister for a few days he is asking for a repeat methadone script. The GP phones for advice about how to manage this patient. Which is the *single* most appropriate management option to suggest? ★

A Arrange a UDS and prescribe methadone if the urine is positive for opiates

B Contact his key worker at the methadone programme to confirm the patient's account

C Prescribe codeine as an alternative to cover the period that he is away from home

D Prescribe methadone 40 mg to be taken supervised by a pharmacist OD

E Refuse to prescribe methadone as it is not possible to prescribe this to a temporary patient

13. A 19-year-old man is diagnosed with OCD. His parents are concerned that other members of the family may go on to develop this diagnosis and so they would like to know more about the condition and how it can be spotted. Which *single* symptom is most likely to be present? ★

A Aggressive thoughts

B Bodily fears

C Checking

D Counting

E Tics

14. A 34-year-old woman has a prolonged episode of low mood for the first time in her life. She describes a four-week mild depressive episode, but she is able to continue working and has maintained good relationships with her friends and family. Which is the *single* most appropriate intervention to offer her? ★

A Amitriptyline

B Citalopram

C Computerized CBT

D Interpersonal therapy (IPT)

E St John's wort

15. A 38-year-old man has been taking citalopram for three months as treatment for a severe depressive episode. He has had no symptoms of depression for one week and would like to know how long he should take the medication for. At this point in time, which is the *single* most appropriate length of time to continue his citalopram? ★

A Stop now

B Two months

C Four months

D Six months

E Eight months

16. A 19-year-old man has reduced concentration and increasing difficulty with his university studies which are causing moderate impairment. He was diagnosed with attention deficit hyperactivity disorder (ADHD) at eight years old but stopped taking medication 18 months ago after finishing his A-levels and travelling in his gap year. He leads an active social life, which includes drinking alcohol, but denies any illicit drugs. Which is the *single* most appropriate management? ★★

A Educational psychologist referral

B Methylphenidate

C Motivational interviewing assessment

D Psychodynamic psychotherapy

E Watchful waiting

17. A 25-year-old woman has a diagnosis of schizophrenia. She has had to be treated in hospital on two occasions and is keen to avoid another admission. She would like to know if there is a psycho-social intervention that is proven to be effective at preventing a relapse requiring hospital admission. Which is the *single* most appropriate initial management? ★★

A Behavioural family therapy

B Computerized CBT

C Exercise

D IPT

E Psychodynamic psychotherapy

18. A 32-year-old woman with BPAD is stable on treatment with lithium. She is keen on having a baby with her partner and is interested to know whether she can continue taking lithium during pregnancy. Which is the *single* most appropriate adverse effect to warn her about? ★★

A Ebstein's anomaly

B Fatal agranulocytosis

C Neonatal haemorrhage

D Neutral tube defects

E Tetralogy of Fallot

19. A 68-year-old woman has received a diagnosis of agoraphobia. Her husband does not understand what this diagnosis means and would like information on what situations she is most likely to avoid. Which is the *single* most appropriate answer to give him? ★★

A Cooking a meal

B Giving a presentation

C Going on a train

D Having a dinner party

E Seeing friends

20. A 45-year-old man has brief periods of chest pain, paraesthesia, and dyspnoea. He is very worried that he has angina. An ECG and troponin taken 12 hours after one episode are both normal. Which is the *single* most appropriate intervention? ★★

A Blood glucose measurement

B Diazepam 10 mg OD for three months

C Echocardiogram

D Explain nothing is wrong

E Self-help book

21. A 56-year-old woman has had several hospital admissions for relapses of BPAD. She has been offered support from her community mental health team (CMHT). She knows there are a wide range of different professionals working there but would like to know which healthcare professionals are not included in this team. Which is the *single* most appropriate answer to give her? ★★

A CPN

B GP

C OT

D Psychologist

E Support worker

22. A 35-year-old man is the victim of a serious assault. He has read on the internet that, after a traumatic event, around 10% of people will develop PTSD. He would like to know what action can increase the likelihood of developing this condition. Which is the *single* most appropriate answer to give him? ★★

A Admission to a psychiatric hospital

B Drinking alcohol

C Having an immediate debriefing session

D Intensive media coverage

E Taking dexamethasone

23. A 46-year-old woman has been experiencing a depressive episode for around one year, but has seen little improvement in her symptoms. She would like to know how likely it is that her depressive episode will last at least another year. She asks the proportion of people who experience symptoms of depression two years after onset. Which is the *single* most appropriate answer to give her? ★★

A 5%

B 15%

C 25%

D 35%

E 45%

24. A PhD student has recently been diagnosed with schizophrenia. He is very upset and states that this will mean there is no point in finishing his degree as he will 'never be able to hold down a proper job'. Which *single* factor predicts a good prognosis at first presentation? ★★

A CMHT input

B High levels of expressed emotion

C Later age of onset

D Male sex

E No stressful precipitant

25. A 27-year-old man had a moderate depressive episode for which he received paroxetine and CBT. He has been without symptoms for 18 months, although he continues to take medication. At his review, he says that he is driving his car to appointments and as part of his job as a salesman. What is the *single* most appropriate initial management regarding his driving? ★★★

A Ask him to inform the Driver and Vehicle Licensing Agency (DVLA)

B Inform the DVLA of his illness

C Notify his insurance provider of his illness

D Seek advice from the local Caldicott Guardian

E Take no action about this situation

26. Knowledge about the burden of mental health problems is vital in making public health decisions about allocating resources. This can be calculated using the number of disability-adjusted life years (DALYs) lost worldwide. A public health doctor is tasked with finding out which psychiatric conditions have the highest worldwide DALYs and to rank them in order. Which *single* condition is most likely to be first in this list? ★★★

A Alcohol use disorders

B BPAD

C Dementia

D Depression (unipolar)

E Schizophrenia

27. A 28-year-old woman has a diagnosis of bulimia nervosa. After Princess Diana discussed having the same condition, the number of people diagnosed with bulimia increased substantially. Which is the *single* most widely accepted explanation for this increase? ★★★

A Copycat behaviour

B Increased expectations to be thin

C Increased health-seeking behaviour

D Mass hysteria

E Overdiagnosis

28. The distribution of mental health conditions in society is important for both allocating resources and understanding risk factors. Although mental illnesses are more common in people currently of a lower socioeconomic status, some are associated with a higher current socioeconomic status. Which *single* mental illness is most likely to be in this category? ★★★

A Alcohol dependency

B BPAD

C Panic disorder

D Schizophrenia

E Unipolar depression

29. A 32-year-old woman experiences two months of hearing a running commentary on her actions and believing that the TV was talking about her. It resolves with treatment. She is very concerned about this happening again and wants to know the likelihood of this being the only episode. Which is the *single* most appropriate approximate answer to give? ★★★

A 0%

B 20%

C 40%

D 60%

E 80%

30. A 23-year-old woman smokes cannabis and has done so for the last three years. She does not feel that this is a problem. Her partner worries about her smoking and has read about change interventions. He asks that you get her to 'stop smoking'. He mentions Prochaska and Diclemente's change cycle. Which *single* stage of this cycle is this woman most likely to be in? ★★★

A Action

B Contemplative

C Maintenance

D Precontemplative

E Preparation

31. A fellow foundation year 1 doctor (FY1) tells you she has been suffering from depression for the last six months. She alleges that the nursing staff are trying to harm her by inserting thoughts into her head. She does not think these experiences are related to her own mental health, but has been seeing a psychiatrist. Which is the *single* most appropriate initial course of action? ★★★

A Call the GMC

B Call the police

C Inform her consultant

D Offer to prescribe her risperidone

E Suggest that she take time off

32. A 45-year-old man has high levels of anxiety. He has done some research about anxiety using the internet and has come to the conclusion that it's a 'women's condition', given that most anxiety disorders are more common in women. He asks if there are any anxiety diagnoses that have an equal distribution between men and women. Which is the *single* most appropriate condition to use as an example? ★★★

A Generalized anxiety disorder

B Mixed anxiety and depression

C OCD

D Panic disorder

E Specific phobia

33. A 26-year-old man has schizophrenia. He wants to know what led to him developing schizophrenia. Several factors have been associated with the development of schizophrenia in case control or cohort studies. Which *single* factor is strongly associated with this? ★★★

A A brother with schizophrenia

B Cannabis use in early teens

C Childhood social difficulties

D Immigrant status

E Obstetric complications

34. A 23-year-old man has difficulties relating to other people. He attends a psychiatric assessment where it is found that, although he does not meet the general criteria for having a PD, he does score highly on a specific questionnaire. Which is the *single* most likely description of his difficulties? ★★★★

A Anankastic PD

B Antisocial PD

C Paranoid PD

D Psychopathy

E Schizoid PD

35. ICD-10 and the Diagnostic and Statistical Manual of Mental Disorders Fifth Edition (DSM–V) include a number of personality disorder (PD) diagnoses. A patient whose partner has just been diagnosed says that this is a way of giving everyone a psychiatric diagnosis and that there is no logic to it. Which *single* answer best describes this approach to personality? ★★★★

A Alienist

B Categorical

C Dimensional

D Ideothetic

E Nomothetic

Extended Matching Questions

Personality disorders

For each patient, chose the single most likely diagnosis from the list of options below. Each option may be used once, more than once, or not at all. ★

A Anankastic PD

B Anxious or avoidant PD

C Dependent PD

D Dissocial PD

E Emotionally unstable PD—borderline type

F Emotionally unstable PD—impulsive type

G Histrionic PD

H No PD/normal personality

I Paranoid PD

J Schizoid PD

1. A 20-year-old woman with changeable mood is dramatic in her description of relationships and conflicts with others. She constantly seeks appreciation and is often the centre of attention. She is distressed because yet another relationship has broken up. She is dressed in a low-cut top and appears to be flirting with another patient in the waiting room.

2. A 25-year-old man with an explosive temper and a tendency to drink to excess has assaulted a man who was talking to his girlfriend. He expressed no concern at the fact that he fractured the jaw of his victim.

3. An 18-year-old man has become increasingly isolated and aloof during his teenage years. He has showed an indifference to the recent death of his grandmother, has no friends, and his only interest seems to be in his collection of Nazi memorabilia.

4. A 23-year-old student is unable to keep up with her course work because she is excessively conscientious to the point that she never completes any of her assignments. She is never satisfied that the quality of her work is good enough and has feelings of doubt about her ability and tends to go over her course material repeatedly.

5. A 23-year-old woman has feelings of depression and listlessness. She relies excessively on other people, first her parents, now her husband. She has a fear that he would leave her because of her behaviour and inability to make simple decisions for herself.

Medication for common conditions

For each scenario below, choose the *single* most appropriate antidepressant from the list of options. Each option may be used once, more than once, or not at all. ★★

A Amitriptyline

B Bupropion

C Citalopram

D Dothiepin

E Fluoxetine

F Flupenthixol

G Mirtazapine

H Moclobemide

I Tranylcypromine

J Venlafaxine

6. A 28-year-old man is suffering from a moderately severe episode of depression. His most prominent symptoms are anhedonia, insomnia, and loss of appetite.

7. A 43-year-old woman working full time has a history of recurrent depression and is currently suffering from a severe episode of depression. She has previously tried citalopram and mirtazapine with little effect.

8. A 19-year-old woman attends the ED following an overdose of her grandmother's antidepressant. She is drowsy and her ECG shows a sinus tachycardia. Collateral history reveals that her grandmother suffers with depression and trigeminal neuralgia.

9. A 53-year-old man with no physical health problems suffers with recurrent depressive disorder, the current episode being severe. He has not derived any lasting benefit from various antidepressants, although citalopram has recently been of some use. His psychiatrist wishes to augment his citalopram with another antidepressant.

10. A 66-year-old man on a long-term antidepressant has a recent onset of severe hypertension. He reports drinking large amounts of red wine since retiring from work recently.

Depressive symptoms

For each presentation, select the *single* most likely diagnosis from the above list of options. Each option may be used once, more than once, or not at all. ★★

A Adjustment disorder

B BPAD

C Cyclothymia

D Depressive pseudodementia

E Dysthymia

F Mild depressive episode

G Moderate depressive episode

H Recurrent depressive disorder

I Severe depressive episode

J Substance misuse

11. A 25-year-old man with low mood has not left his home for two months as he has lost interest in his usual hobbies. He is eating less and has lost 5 kg. He tells his sister that he feels helpless, a burden to the family, and his future seems hopeless.

12. A 28-year-old woman has had low mood, lack of energy, and sleep disturbance for two months. She has had two similar episodes in the past five years. She has been drinking heavily for a month. She has a history of mood swings and in between the low episodes she is full of energy and tends to overspend.

13. A 58-year-old publican has had low mood for six months. Recently he has become increasingly anxious and irritable and finds it difficult to concentrate on running his business. He has reddened palms and numerous blanching red spots on his chest.

14. A 15-year-old adolescent is no longer interested in hockey when she had previously been the best player on the school team. Her mother is worried that for the past seven months she has been withdrawn, sleeping poorly, and has lost a lot of weight. The young person denies any appetite loss.

15. A 46-year-old woman has experienced mood swings since her early twenties. She feels she is constantly either high or low and feels this affects her ability to work, although she does not miss more than a couple of days' work at a time. When feeling high she becomes restless and talkative. When feeling low she experiences tearfulness and poor sleep. She finds that alcohol and drugs have allowed her to self-medicate, but she does not use these outside of the episodes.

ANSWERS

Single Best Answers

1. A ★   OHPsych 3rd edn → pp. 495, 758–9

Asperger's syndrome is the most likely diagnosis (A). The classic diagnostic triad is difficulties in reciprocal social interaction, communication, and restricted, stereotyped, repetitive behaviour. Language delay or cognitive impairment would lead to a diagnosis of autism. Asperger's syndrome was removed in DSM-V and replaced with 'high functioning austism spectrum disorder'.

For a diagnosis of autism (B) there must be evidence of language delay before the age of three years old. Autism is considered to be part of a spectrum of behaviours affecting a person's social and communication abilities. Asperger's syndrome is also on this spectrum, but people with this diagnosis tend to be 'higher functioning'.

An intelligence quotient (IQ) less than 70 is required for a diagnosis of learning disability. While people allege A-levels have been dumbed down, it is unlikely this man has a mild learning difficulty (LD) (C) if he passed two.

People with paranoid PD (D) can avoid other people, but this avoidance is mainly due to misinterpreting other's actions as threatening. Sexual relationships are often characterized by recurrent worries about their partner's fidelity.

This is often called schizotypal PD (E) as it combines some psychosis-like symptoms with lifelong personality traits of difficulties establishing and maintaining relationships with other people. Fragmentary psychotic experiences characterize this condition, which has an uncertain relationship to schizophrenia; however, there are no such experiences mentioned here.

→ ICD-10: http://apps.who.int/classifications/icd10/browse/2010/en.

2. D ★   OHPsych 3rd edn → pp.54–5, 358–9, 364–78

Recurrent panic attacks, which can occur in different situations, are consistent with panic disorder (D). A panic attack usually begins abruptly and includes rapid heartbeat or palpitations, shortness of breath, sweating, dizziness, tingling, and severe 'anxiousness'. A person experiencing these may assume that they are in acute physical danger of a heart attack or something similar and report feeling as though they might die. This only serves to increase the anxiety and make the symptoms worse, creating a vicious cycle.

Agoraphobia (A) is the fear of certain places, usually where escape may be difficult, for example trains or busy spaces, and of large crowds. Its root is from the Greek 'αγορά' (agro) meaning 'gathering place'. Often people with this diagnosis show great anticipatory anxiety—getting worried before the event, leading to avoidance of the situation. It is the most common phobia seen by psychiatrists.

There are no clear symptoms of depression (B) in this clinical scenario and so it is not possible to make the diagnosis from this. Anxiety and panic attacks can occur with depressive symptoms, but this is not the most likely diagnosis here.

No obsessions or compulsions are described in this clinical scenario, making this diagnosis very unlikely. There can be many different emotions experienced in OCD (C), including upset, panic, and depression.

In social phobia (E) the anxiety is related to specific situations, such as being in a public place or a stressful situation, having to engage with other people, or having to actively participate in the situation. It would be highly unlikely that someone would experience an episode of social phobia while watching the television.

→ RCPsych information on anxiety, panic and phobias: http://www.rcpsych.ac.uk/expertadvice/problemsdisorders/anxietyphobiaskeyfacts.aspx.

→ YouTube video of embarrassing bodies—panic attack: http://www.youtube.com/watch?v=0qfHboZqN7I.

3. C ★   OHPsych 3rd edn → pp.248–9

Five percent of people with depression have clinically significant hypothyroidism (C). Other symptoms include weight gain, decreased sweating, changes in menstruation, and bradycardia.

Glioma (A) is a rare condition, but symptoms include headaches, nausea and vomiting, seizures, and low mood.

Hypercalcaemia (B) is associated with 'stones (renal or bilary), bones (pain), groans (abdominal pain and depression)'.

Sleep apnoea (D) may present with lethargy, low mood, and poor motivation but will be accompanied by characteristic sleep abnormalities.

Both exogenous and endogenous excess steroids can lead to mood disturbances and psychotic symptoms. 'Roid rage' is a lay term for the changes in personality often seen when athletes take steroids, but less than 1% of the population take steroids regularly (E).

→ Gold MS, Pottash AL, Extein I (1981). Hypothyroidism and depression: evidence from complete thyroid function evaluation. *Journal of the American Medical Association*, **245** (19), 1919–22.

4. C ★   OHPsych 3rd edn → pp.398–408

The answer is bulimia nervosa (C). A binge is defined as a period of overeating, usually of high carbohydrate foods. During a binge people feel like they have lost control of their eating and then feel guilty after. In bulimia this is accompanied by a fear of fatness and efforts to reduce the effect of calories consumed. Inducing vomiting, using diet pills or laxatives, or exercise are common ways to attempt to prevent weight gain after a binge.

A pathological fear of fatness, efforts to reduce weight, and, crucially for this question, a BMI less than 17.5 kg/m² (with subsequent metabolic changes) would lead to diagnosis of anorexia (A). Binges are a common part of anorexia but BMI is the key differentiating sign between the two main eating disorders.

Pathological fear of fatness is not part of binge eating disorder (B). Most sufferers are overweight with a BMI of over 30 kg/m². The difference between this and bulimia is that people who binge eat do not purge themselves afterwards to make a direct effort to control their weight. They tend to limit their weight gain by stopping eating, or having very little, outside of the binges. This often leads to more binges, weight gain, and ultimately obesity.

While the fear of gaining weight in both anorexia nervosa and bulimia nervosa can approach delusional intensity, the characteristic behaviour described makes delusional disorder very unlikely (D).

Again, fear of fatness would not be associated with elite training (E) and the goal of being a specific weight is related to the specific demands of the sport. There have been high-profile athletes, such as GB triathlon world champion Hollie Avil, who have developed an eating disorder which forced them to quit training entirely. In any situation where there is a pressure to reach and keep a certain body shape and weight there is an increased danger of an eating disorder developing, and some crossover of endocrine changes, but there still needs to be a the clinical psychological signs for a diagnosis to be made.

→ ICD-10: http://apps.who.int/classifications/icd10/browse/2010/en#/F50-F59.

5. E ★　　OHPsych 3rd edn → pp.358–9, 364–78

Social phobia is the most common of these anxiety disorders with a prevalence of 7.9% (E). A household survey is described by the Government as 'an interdepartmental multipurpose continuous survey carried out by the Office for National Statistics collecting information on a range of topics from people living in private households in Great Britain'.

From Harvard Medical School's National Comorbidity Survey the figure for agoraphobia (A) is around 2.8–5.8%. This makes it less common in prevalence than social phobia, but, as we have seen in an earlier question, it is the most common phobia seen by psychiatrists as people with it tend to seek help rather than ignore it. This might be because its symptoms are more obvious and life-limiting.

Around 2.5–6.4% of people in the survey met the criteria for a diagnosis of generalized anxiety disorder (B). By comparison, the prevalence of epilepsy in the UK is also around 6.2% (according to the GP register). It is helpful to be able to put the disorders in the context of other 'common' conditions so that the diagnosis appears less frightening.

The quoted figure of 0.5–2% makes OCD (C) always the lowest in prevalence of these conditions. It is important to consider both prevalence and impact when considering a diagnosis and the reasons that someone may be seeking help.

The figure of 4.2% is given for the prevalence of panic disorders (D) in the population. While it is not essential to know the exact prevalence of every disorder, it is helpful to be able to consider which are more common and to be able to translate these into information for patients and their families. For example, being able to say that 'on average there will be at least another three people with this condition living in your block of 100 people' makes the diagnosis less stigmatizing.

→ National Comorbidity Survey: http://www.hcp.med.harvard.edu/ncs/index.php.

6. A ★ OHPsych 3rd edn → pp.404–5

The need for inpatient care is largely driven by the medical complications of very low weight. Hypothermia (body temperature 35.5°C) (A) is an indication that weight stabilization in hospital is urgently needed and thus is the correct answer.

While difficult family dynamics (B) are often cited as an aetiological factor in developing anorexia, it is not a reason alone for inpatient care. Family therapy is often a component of the management of anorexia.

While there is limited evidence that antidepressants alter the course of anorexia itself, people with anorexia suffer high rates of depression and suicide. There is no requirement for antidepressants to be started in hospital (C).

'Pro-ana' refers to the promotion of very low body weight as a lifestyle choice, rather than an illness (D). It is based on a shortening of 'pro-anorexia', with 'pro-mia' focusing on bulimia. While having these views may indicate poor engagement with care, starting a blog would not be a key factor in determining the need for inpatient care.

Using diet pills (E) is not a key factor in determining the need for inpatient care. However, it is important to bear in mind that many diet pills contain amphetamine, especially those sourced from the Americas. This can lead to the development of a psychotic illness, which would lead to the consideration of inpatient care.

→ Bond E (2012). *Virtually anorexic—where's the harm? A research study on the risks of pro-anorexia websites.* www.ucs.ac.uk/virtuallyanorexic.

7. E ★ OHPsych 3rd edn → pp.56–7, 95–103

The answer is reflex hallucinations (E). These occur when a sensory input in one modality (in this case, the car horns) causes a hallucination in another modality (the visual hallucination of fireworks). Reflex hallucinations are often experienced under the influence of psychedelic drugs; however, after repeated use, some users may experience flashbacks—spontaneous recurrences of illusions and visual hallucinations during the drug-free state. This phenomenon can occur months after the last drug use.

Command hallucinations (A) are hallucinations where the patient experiences being given a command; these are usually auditory or within their mind. They may range from simple harmless orders to commands of significant violence towards themselves or others. They are commonly associated with schizophrenia.

Elementary hallucinations (B) are hallucinations of low complexity, such as hearing ringing, rustling, or buzzing noises. Auditory hallucinations where voices or music are heard would be classified as complex hallucinations, rather than elementary ones.

Extracampine hallucinations (C) occur outside the field of normal perception, for example hearing voices from beyond the range of possible hearing distance.

Gedankenlautwerden (D) refers to complex auditory hallucinations where a patient hears thoughts spoken aloud in the form of a voice. Unlike thought echo, these voices are heard at the same time they are thought, rather than directly afterwards.

→ Chaudhury S (2010). Hallucinations: clinical aspects and management. *Industrial Psychiatry Journal*, **19** (1), 5–12.

8. C ★   OHPsych 3rd edn → pp.376–8

The answer is OCD (C). This is characterized by obsessional thoughts and compulsions that interfere with functioning (social, educational) and cause distress. He is unable to complete tasks due to the repetitive nature of the compulsions.

Although there have been some important life events, for example a new job in a new place, these aren't directly linked to his symptoms, so an adjustment disorder is not an appropriate diagnosis (A).

His beliefs don't appear delusional in nature and his awareness of the thoughts being 'odd' makes an early-onset psychosis unlikely (B). It is always difficult to ascertain with any certainty that a belief is delusional without proper assessment. From personal experience, a patient who tells you they have recently spoken to the Queen at Buckingham Palace may actually have done so—so do not judge too quickly.

There is no evidence in the scenario that he has panic attacks or periods of acute anxiety (D). While he is clearly worried about a number of things, these are better explained in the context of OCD.

PTSD (E) can be confused with OCD due to the avoidance and unusual behaviour. However, it would require a life-endangering event prior to the symptoms starting and subsequent changes in sleep pattern, nightmares, and hypervigilance.

→ OCDAction: http://www.ocdaction.org.uk/.

→ YouTube video about understanding OCD (by OCD-UK): https://www.youtube.com/watch?v=_YOcjtEzgHs.

9. A ★   OHPsych 3rd edn → pp.190–3, 196–7

Early intervention services (A) have been set up to provide specialist care for people in the early stages of a psychotic illness. They aim to moderate the long-term course of schizophrenia by targeting the period of the illness where the most functional loss occurs: the first two years. Whether this can be changed specifically by an early intervention service remains controversial, and many people argue that evidence-based care should be provided to everyone with schizophrenia, rather than a specific group.

There is no evidence that general hospital care is needed in this case (B). Disorientation, neurological signs, or serious substance withdrawal may indicate the need for care in a general hospital.

Although GPs are very used to managing patients with mental health problems (C), care of psychosis, especially early in the illness, should be provided by specialist mental health services where possible.

With a supportive family, willingness to engage with services, and no serious risk identified, inpatient psychiatric care is not indicated (D).

Rehabilitation services (E) focus on the approximately 15% of people with schizophrenia who continue to have symptoms despite normal psychiatric care. This proportion has not been changed by early intervention services.

→ NICE Clinical Guideline 82—Schizophrenia: http://www.nice.org. uk/CG82.

10. B ★   OHPsych 3rd edn → pp.362–3

Seven to 14 hours of CBT (B) is the most effective treatment for panic disorder according to NICE guidance. This is considered to be the first-line treatment, and further consideration of the diagnosis and alternative treatment should be considered if no significant change in symptoms results from this intervention alone.

Amitriptyline 75 mg OD is not an effective anxiolytic and is not recommended, although its sedative side-effects can lead to people reporting a reduction in levels of agitation (A).

While as-required benzodiazepines (e.g. diazepam 5 mg OD) (C) can be useful to reduce acute levels of anxiety, regular use for more than two weeks is not indicated. This has been shown to lead to a poorer prognosis.

Flooding (D) is an old-fashioned behavioural approach to phobias. While flooding has been shown to be as effective as a structured, graded approach to the extinction of phobia, the experience is not as well tolerated by patients and results in increased disengagement with treatment. Flooding can be done in the patient's imagination rather than by physical exposure, in which case it is called 'implosion'.

Self-help (E) has been shown to be beneficial for mild anxiety disorders, but it is not as effective as CBT. If a patient is not willing to commit to the diagnosis or the treatment, then suggesting an appropriate self-help book, or website, can destigmatize the diagnosis and promote engagement. The Royal College of Psychiatry website has a factsheet with useful suggestions for each condition.

→ NICE Clinical Guideline 113—Anxiety: http://guidance.nice.org.uk/CG113.

→ RCPsych information on problem disorders: http://www.rcpsych.ac.uk/healthadvice/problemsdisorders.aspx.

11. C ★   OHPsych 3rd edn → pp.968–71

Olanzapine (C) is not thought to cause congenital malformations or miscarriage, but data are limited in this regard. It may be associated with large-for-gestational-age babies. It would be the most appropriate prophylaxis medication as it has the least known teratogenic effects.

Carbamezapine (A) is associated with a 1% rate of neural tube defects, as well as heart defects and hypospadias.

Lithium use in pregnancy (B) is teratogenic, associated with a 4–12% rate of major congenital malformations and an increased miscarriage risk. Its use in pregnancy increases the risk of Ebstein's anomaly (a malformation of the tricuspid valve) by tenfold.

Paroxetine (D) is associated with ventricular septal defects, cleft lip, and palate and digestive system abnormalities (imperforate anus, pyloric stenosis).

Like carbamezapine, sodium valproate (E) is an antiepileptic associated with increased risk of neural tube defects, heart defects, and hypospadias, and also causes skeletal abnormalities. The overall risk of malformation is higher with sodium valproate than carbamezapine.

12. B ★   OHPsych 3rd edn → pp.596–9

Getting confirmation of the patient's account is very important before any prescription is issued (B). The GP may want to check whether the patient is known to the methadone service, when they were last seen, what their maintenance dose is, and whether they are on supervised doses. GPs may feel under pressure from an angry, distressed, or withdrawing patient to believe their account and prescribe immediately, but without verifying the information there could be serious, or even fatal, consequences.

Although the positive urine screen indicates that the patient does take opiates it will not give any confirmation of dose (A). Even though the patient is not opiate-naïve, it could be dangerous to prescribe methadone if he is not actually taking it already, or if he is taking a lower dose than he says. It is imperative to check the background information before prescribing methadone to this patient. If he is not methadone-tolerant, taking this may lead to fatal respiratory depression. Also patients on opiate replacement therapies should be part of a structured drug recovery and rehabilitation programme.

Codeine is not licensed for use in drug dependence, although it may rarely be used by specialists when patients are taking street dihydrocodeine, or in the final stages of methadone reduction. It should not be used as an alternative to methadone prescription in this situation (C).

Patients have died from overdoses when well-meaning clinicians have prescribed methadone without checking first whether the patient is in a supervised opiate replacement programme. The patient should not be prescribed methadone without (ideally written) confirmation of the dose he is taking from a member of staff from the methadone service (D).

Prescribing methadone may be possible even if he is registered as a temporary patient. The GP should certainly not be obstructive (E) and should try to help the patient by offering to contact their methadone service prior to issuing a prescription.

→ NICE Technology Appraisal 114—Methadone and buprenorphine for managing opioid dependence: http://www.nice.org.uk/ta114.

---

13. C ★ OHPsych 3rd edn → pp.376–8

Using the Yale–Brown Obsessive Compulsive Scale (YBOCS) the many symptoms of OCD can be assessed. Checking is the most common symptom reported in OCD: by two-thirds of people (C). The checking ritual that is present can be checking for something physical, such as an unlocked door or iron left turned on, or a worry, such as harm coming to a loved one (frequently ringing them to check) or a stranger (scouring the news for stories).

Aggressive thoughts (A) are reported by a quarter of people with OCD. They are very unlikely to be acted on and are usually resisted; however, the frequency and horrible nature of the thoughts and mental images can be very disturbing—and often the person having these believes that they must harbour a dislike of the recipient, otherwise they would not get them. This isn't the case.

One-third of people with OCD report worries about their body's func-tion, including hypochondriacal fears (B). There is a crossover with a checking ritual where the person makes sure that they aren't developing a medical condition—thereafter checking their pulse or blood pressure (BP) all the time.

One-third of people with OCD report counting as a symptom (D). Often the counting rituals will involve doing something a certain number of times, in multiples of a certain number, or the avoidance of a number. All this can leave a person with OCD distracted and unable to complete tasks.

People with Tourette's syndrome are more likely to have OCD, but it is a rare condition. Tics (E) are defined as rapid, repetitive, involuntary contractions of a group of muscles.

→ Yale–Brown Obsessive Compulsive Scale: http://www.mssm.edu/research/centers/center-of-excellence-for-ocd/rating-scales.

---

14. C ★ OHPsych 3rd edn → pp.252–3

Both computerized CBT (C) and guided self-help using CBT approaches are recommended by NICE for the treatment of a mild episode. A group-based exercise programme is also recommended, but watchful waiting (review about every two weeks) would also be an option based on patient choice.

Antidepressants such as amitriptyline (A) do not differentiate from placebo until the patient has at least a moderate depressive episode. The depression severity, according to DSM-IV, can be made based on the number of symptoms and the impairment these have on the person. Therefore, subthreshold depressive episodes have fewer than five symptoms, and a mild depression diagnosis is made where there are just five symptoms required to make the diagnosis and only minor functional impairment. Severe depression is where all symptoms are seen and these markedly interfere with functioning. Severe depression can occur with or without psychotic symptoms.

As previously described, antidepressants (such as citalopram) (B) do not differentiate from placebo until the patient has at least a moderate depressive episode.

IPT (D) focuses on the patient's interpersonal network as a way to improve their mental health. It is an effective treatment for depression, but it is not recommended for a mild depressive episode.

St John's wort (E) does lead to a significantly greater reduction in depressive symptoms than placebo, but the immense variability of preparations and its interactions with other drugs mean that it is not recommended for use as an antidepressant.

→ NICE Clinical Guideline 90—Depression in adults: quick reference guide: http://guidance.nice.org.uk/CG90/QuickRefGuide/pdf/English.

---

15. D ★   OHPsych 3rd edn → pp.256–7

An antidepressant should be taken for at least six months after resolution of the symptoms (D). In randomized controlled trials (RCTs) around 50% of people will see a recurrence of the depressive episode if the treatment is stopped before six months. In this case, the patient has seen a resolution after three months so should end up taking antidepressant medication for a total of nine months, but in another patient it could be after four months (totalling ten months) or six months (totalling 12 months).

There is clear evidence of a return of symptoms if antidepressants are stopped too early (A). As only two-thirds of patients actually request enough prescriptions to complete the course, let alone actually take the tablets, the impact of stopping too early on the prevalence of depression may be large.

Stopping after too short a period of symptom resolution (e.g. two months) (B) increases the risk of recurrence. Six months is the recommended duration for this man to continue his citalopram course.

Again, four months (C) is shorter than the recommended time frame and may increase his risk of recurrence.

Longer durations of treatment may be recommended if the patient has had recurrent episodes of depression (E).

→ NICE Clinical Guideline 90—Depression in adults: http://guidance. nice.org.uk/CG90.

16. B ★★ OHPsych 3rd edn → pp.628–9

Given that ADHD has been diagnosed and he has previously shown a good response to this, it would be most appropriate to restart the medication and monitor his behaviour (B). As with any use of methylphenidate, appropriate initial investigations should be completed before restarting the medication, and a maintenance regime plan should be agreed with the patient. Adult ADHD is a widely accepted diagnosis, with a rough guideline being that approximately a third of children with ADHD no longer have symptoms by age 18, one-third have some symptoms which are manageable without medication, and about a third require a regular prescription. There is variability in the diagnosis of ADHD across the world which suggests that there is a strong cultural component to its diagnosis and treatment.

Educational psychologists (A) are useful in determining the probable cause of educational difficulties—for example, inability to concentrate in class or underperformance in an academic setting—and referring on to the appropriate professional or offering situational support. However, in this case a diagnosis has already been made for ADHD and therefore it is a matter of how best to manage the symptoms of this.

Motivational interviewing (C) is most frequently used to help people change their problematic behaviours. This is often due to addiction to drugs or alcohol. In this case the difficulties in behaviour are due to ADHD and there is no evidence of a drug or alcohol problem. Methylphenidate is not advised where there is illicit drug use, so, were this present and were it preventing a prescription, motivational interviewing could be considered first to help stop the drug use, with medication to follow when drug-free.

Psychotherapy is not considered of use in ADHD (D). There is evidence to suggest that a behavioural therapeutic approach can be of use, but this tends to be CBT, or something that has a clear behaviour-focused goal, and used in conjunction with medication.

These behaviours are clearly causing a moderate degree of impairment to this man's education. There is no reason to avoid treating such a problem if there is an evidence-based treatment available (E). Assuming he was willing to take medication, there is help available to allow him to maximize his potential at universality and avoid his ADHD causing him to fail to achieve better grades.

→ NICE Clinical Guideline 72—Attention deficit hyperactivity disorder: diagnosis and management of ADHD in children, young people and adults: http://publications.nice.org.uk/attention-deficit-hyperactivity-disorder-cg72.

17. A ★★ OHPsych 3rd edn → pp.198–9

There is clear evidence that behavioural family therapy (A) reduces hospital admission by improving family communication, problem solving, and reducing expressed emotion.

Face-to-face CBT reduces the risk of symptomatic relapse but has not been shown to have a consistent effect at reducing hospital admission. Computerized CBT has not been shown to be effective in psychosis (B).

Exercise (C) has wider benefits but has not been linked to reducing hospital admission. Therefore, it would be sensible to promote exercise in general and to talk about its beneficial qualities in maintaining mental health, but this is not the initial treatment choice.

IPT (D) has not been evaluated in psychosis. Early trials are currently in progress. This answer may be updated in later editions based on the new evidence (or not, depending on statistical significance).

There is no evidence that psychodynamic psychotherapy is effective at reducing hospital admission (E). Moreover, there are no large clinical trials for this at this time.

→ NICE Clinical Guideline 82— Schizophrenia: http://www.nice.org.uk/CG82.

18. A ★★   OHPsych 3rd edn → pp.968–9

Ebstein's anomaly (A) is a congenital cardiac defect where the septal leaflet of the tricuspid valve is displaced towards the apex of the right ventricle. It accounts for less than 1% of all congenital cardiac cases. The risk is increased in women taking lithium in pregnancy, and so this potential adverse effect should be discussed with the patient.

Numerous medications cause agranulocytosis, including carbamezapine, antithyroid medications, and clozapine. Patients who take clozapine are monitored for this adverse effect by having regular FBC tests. Lithium is not associated with fatal agranulocytosis (B).

Lithium does not affect coagulation pathways. It does not cause bleeding side-effects in patients or in newborns exposed to lithium during pregnancy (C).

Neural tube defects (D) are associated with antiepileptic medications, such as carbamezapine, sodium valproate, and phenytoin, and other folate antagonists, such as trimethoprim. If a woman takes antiepileptic medication during pregnancy she should also take high-dose folic acid (5 mg per day, compared with the usual 400 micrograms per day) to reduce the risk of neural tube defects.

Tetralogy of Fallot (E) is a congenital cardiac defect where there is a ventricular septal defect, overriding aorta, right ventricular outflow obstruction, and consequently right ventricular hypertrophy. It may be associated with genetic conditions but is not associated with the use of medications in pregnancy.

→ Attenhofer Jost CH, Connolly HM, Dearani JA, Edwards WD, Danielson GK (2007). Ebstein's anomaly. *Circulation*, **115** (2), 277–85.

19. C ★★   OHPsych 3rd edn → pp.366–71

The most common fear in agoraphobia is being trapped or unable to escape busy places. Buses, trains (C), and the London Underground are commonly avoided in agoraphobia. ICD-10 defines agoraphobia as: 'A fairly well-defined cluster of phobias embracing fears of leaving home, entering shops, crowds and public places, or travelling alone in trains, buses or planes. Depressive and obsessional symptoms and social phobias are also commonly present as subsidiary features. Avoidance of the phobic situation is often prominent, and some ago-raphobics experience little anxiety because they are able to avoid their phobic situations.'

Cooking a meal (A) is not the most appropriate answer. Worries about eating or of vomiting in front of people are more related to social pho-bia. Fear of vomiting is also known as emetophobia and can restrict a person's life as they cannot go out to eat, travel, or watch certain films because they fear these may induce the vomiting.

Anxiety about performing in small groups is diagnostic of social phobia. If the situation was avoided due to where it was, that would more likely be agoraphobia. Thus, giving a presentation (B) is not appropriate.

Neither is having a dinner party (D). Concerns about eating in front of people are usually seen in social phobia. Often the manner in which people cope with this fear is through avoidance and social isolation or through maladaptive coping strategies such as drinking to excess.

Anxiety around friends (E) tends to be most common in social phobias. Here people are concerned about embarrassing themselves in front of people that they like.

→ ICD-10:

http://apps.who.int/classifications/icd10/browse/2010/en#/
F40-F48.

20. E ★★   OHPsych 3rd edn → pp.22–263

The answer is a self-help book (E). NICE recommends this approach to help people with panic attacks. Self-help books can also be called 'bibliotherapy' and should now include websites and online resources as well as published books. The Royal College of Psychiatrists, amongst others, has a useful list of appropriate books at the end of their patient education leaflets.

These symptoms are highly suggestive of panic attacks. NICE clearly advises that further cardiovascular investigations such as blood glucose measurement (A) are not indicated once a diagnosis of anxiety is made. A thyroid function test should be considered.

Regular benzodiazepines for more than two weeks have been found to be harmful in the long term. The risk of dependence is high with all benzodiazepines. Thus diazepam 10 mg OD for three months would not be appropriate (B).

As this is likely to be a panic attack an echocardiogram (C) would add nothing to this picture. Putting the patient through unnecessary investiga-tions is time consuming, expensive, and can be psychologically damaging.

Patients with panic attacks are often told 'it's all in your head' or 'there is noth-ing wrong' (D). This is unhelpful and can lead to people disengaging with care.

→ NICE Clinical Guideline 113—Anxiety: http://guidance.nice.org.uk/CG113.

21. B ★★ OHPsych 3rd edn → pp.322–3

CMHTs provide secondary-level care. GPs would not be part of the team, although liaison with them is vital to provide good mental health-care across the population. Therefore (B) is the correct answer.

CPNs (A) are always members of the CMHT. CPNs are fully trained psychiatric nurses who have several years' experience working in a psychiatric hospital or ward. They are often patients' key workers within the National Health Service (NHS) mental health system and are often the first port of call for further referrals to psychiatrists, psychotherapists, and other mental health professionals. CPNs mainly visit people in their own homes, but they also see people in other settings such as GP surgeries or at the CMHT base.

The role of the OT (C) is to help each patient achieve a fulfilled and satisfied state in life through the use of 'purposeful activity or interventions designed to achieve functional outcomes which promote health, prevent injury or disability and which develop, improve, sustain or restore the highest possible level of independence'. This is true in mental health as well as for physical health needs.

Psychologists (D) are key members of the CMHT team; often well-developed teams have senior consultant psychologists who can offer expert opinion about new management options and research developments.

Support workers (E) work in CMHTs and tend to work both in the clinic and within non-healthcare settings to better engagement with patients. Their role involves support for health, mental health, and social needs.

→ RCPsych information on mental health services/teams in the community: http://www.rcpsych.ac.uk/expertadvice/treatmentswellbeing/mentalhealthinthecommunity.aspx.

22. C ★★ OHPsych 3rd edn → pp.390–3

There is clear evidence that a debriefing session, where people are encouraged to talk through what happened increases the risk of PTSD (C).

No causal link has been established with PTSD and psychiatric admission (A).

Small cohort studies suggest that moderate alcohol use may be protective, but the evidence is not strong enough for this to be a recommendation (B). Harmful use or dependency on sedative substances often occurs along with PTSD.

No link is established between media coverage and PTSD (D). There is an ongoing debate about whether watching traumatic events, e.g. the terrorist attack on the Twin Towers in New York, can precipitate PTSD in some people.

Patients on intensive treatment units (ITUs) have high rates of PTSD on recovery. One small study of patients who had been on ITU found that regular dexamethasone halved the number of people reporting PTSD symptoms (E). This may be due to the negative feedback effects of steroids on monoamine release.

→ Rose S, Bisson J, Churchill R, Wessely S (2002). Psychological debriefing for preventing post-traumatic stress disorder (PTSD). *Cochrane Database of Systematic Reviews*, (2), CD00056.

23. B ★★   OHPsych 3rd edn → pp.243, 250

Studies estimate that 10–20% of people will continue to experience symptoms at two years (B). As with any question such as this there will always be individual studies that give a different percentage (for example, in a subgroup of people), but it is important to know what the 'official' rates are for incidence, replace, etc. so that you can appropriately inform a patient of the likely prognosis of a disorder. The best way to do this is to look at the Royal College of Psychiatrist's published material or a good, updated textbook (such as the OHPsych!)

The figure of 5% is too low for this question (A). There is good evidence that with modern detection and treatments of depression there will be a significant decrease in reoccurrence rates and that, in the future, chronicity will be as low as 5%.

Approximately 25% of people will have symptoms at one year, but this number will drop when considering symptoms after two years (C).

The figure of 35% (D) is too high for depressive symptoms after two years, although the risk of reoccurrence of depression is approximately 30% at ten years and 60% at 20 years, which suggests that she may well have a second episode at some point in her life.

Forty-five percent (E) is closer to the lifetime risk of experiencing a mental disorder, with nearly half of Americans (46.4%) reported to meet criteria at some point in their life for a DSM-IV anxiety disorder (28.8%), mood disorder (20.8%), impulse-control disorder (24.8%), or substance use disorders (14.6%). Half of all lifetime cases had started by age 14 and three-quarters by age 24.

→ RCPsych information on depression: http://www.rcpsych.ac.uk/ expertadvice/problemsdisorders/depression.aspx.

→ Kessler RC, Berglund P, Demler O, Jin R, Merikangas KR, Walters EE (2005). Lifetime prevalence and age-of-onset distributions of DSM-IV disorders in the National Comorbidity Survey Replication. *Archives of General Psychiatry*, 62 (6), 593–602.

24. C ★★   OHPsych 3rd edn → pp.188–9, 198–9

Later age of onset (C) is a good prognostic sign. The average age of onset is 18 in men and 26 in women. In general, schizophrenia is a disease that typically begins in early adulthood. There is thought to be a falling incidence with age, but this could be due to unreported prodromal/psychotic episodes being undetected due to lack of appropriate diagnostic criteria.

There is no RCT evidence regarding CMHT involvement (A). There is anecdotal evidence, and common sense, to suggest that a positive attitude toward an MDT approach and engaging with help will mean a better outcome overall—although this is confounded by those with co-morbid conditions finding it harder to work with this approach and also having greater difficulties in general.

High expressed emotion (B) describes family members, carers, or professionals who are both blaming and critical towards a person with schizophrenia, and each other. It is associated with a poor prognosis, although it can be significantly modified with behavioural family therapy.

Being a man is associated with a worse prognosis (D). This is partly due to men developing schizophrenia earlier than women, although the average lifetime incidence is equal.

A slow, insidious onset with no clear precipitant (E) is associated with a poor prognosis. This may be due to a longer period of untreated psychosis, or may reflect a worse underlying illness.

→ Bebbington P, Kuipers L (1994). The predictive utility of expressed emotion in schizophrenia: an aggregate analysis. *Psychological Medicine*, **24** (3), 707–18.

25. E ★★★ OHPsych 3rd edn → pp.902–6

The answer is to take no action about this situation (E). The DVLA does not need to know about his condition: he doesn't need to tell them, and nor does the doctor. There are a number of these conditions of relevance to psychiatry, including anorexia, epilepsy, OCD, and dementia, but it must be clear that driving is negatively affected by their medical condition. The DVLA does not need to be notified of a diagnosis of mild or moderate depression, which is controlled, and which does not have somatic symptoms.

There is no reason to inform the DVLA and therefore no reason to request that he does so (A). If he were to have any ongoing symptoms of depression or any associated psychopathology then it would be appropriate to consider who needs to take responsibility for letting the DVLA know about the situation. This is summarized by the DVLA as 'severe anxiety or depression with significant memory and concentration problems, agitation, behavioural disturbance or suicidal thoughts'. If he did need to contact the DVLA it would mean filling in an accurate medical questionnaire and giving consent for the DVLA's doctors to contact the appropriate doctor.

The DVLA requests that it is informed if there is a 'notifiable' medical condition or disability, a worsening of that medical condition, or a new medical condition (B). The DVLA will decide if there needs to a revocation of the licence, a shorter-period licence, or an adaptation of the patient's car by fitting special controls.

As part of the Road Traffic Act (1998) there is a duty for those whose performance is impaired, through mental illness, medication, or any other condition, to inform their insurance company (C). Failure to do this would be considered as 'withholding a material fact' which would mean that they are driving without proper insurance (illegal), and also it would make the insurance policy void and there would be no payout in the event of an accident. In this case, however, such a condition is not present.

Caldicott Guardians (D) are employed by the NHS with a responsibility to ensure patient data are kept secure and to manage how confidential patient information is handled. They must adhere to the six Caldicott principles which include justifying the purpose of the use of patient information, minimizing identifiable information, and making sure everyone is aware of the responsibilities to the patient and the law.

→ DVLA advice on health conditions and driving: https://www.gov.uk/health-conditions-and-driving.

26. D ★★★   OHPsych 3rd edn → pp.232–5, 250

Depression (unipolar) is the highest in this list (D): third of all conditions worldwide and first in high-income countries. While depression is generally treatable, it has a very high prevalence.

Alcohol use disorders is 17th of all conditions worldwide, fifth in high-income countries (A).

Mental disorders are an important source of lost years of healthy life for women aged 15–44 years. They make up three of the ten leading causes of disease burden. Within this, unipolar depression accounts for approximately 20% and bipolar for approximately 5% (B).

Almost 85% of DALYs involved people aged under 59 years. It is important in these questions to consider the worldwide population and the impact on death rates prior to ages where dementia would be prevalent (C).

Schizophrenia (E) is ranked more than 20th in the WHO table. This accounts for approximately 1% of worldwide DALYs, compared to depression which is 4.3%.

→ WHO Global burden of disease 2004: http://www.who.int/healthinfo/global_burden_disease/2004_report_update/en/index.html.

27. C ★★★   OHPsych 3rd edn → pp.6–8

Diagnosis requires a patient to present to a doctor. Increased health-seeking behaviour (C) played the largest part in the increase in diagnoses. Men are particularly poor in terms of health-seeking behaviour, which may influence the reported gender differences in certain disorders.

While it is likely that increasing awareness will have led to some increase in the behaviours described, copycat behaviour (A) is not the major contributor to the large increase in diagnosis. Community studies do not suggest a large increase in prevalence associated with the interview with Martin Bashir for the BBC's *Panorama* programme in 1995.

Increased expectations to be thin (B) is a wider cultural trend which cannot be considered related to a single person or event. That said, certain 'high-profile' cases will encourage others to seek help or to persuade others to look for a diagnosis in family members.

In lay language, hysteria refers to overwhelming excessive outbursts of emotion. Hysteria is an outdated medical diagnosis. It was thought to be a neurotic condition affecting women and to be caused by uterine disturbances ('hystera' is Greek for 'womb'). Thus mass hysteria (D) is not the right answer.

Neither is overdiagnosis (E). Eating disorders remain poorly identified in primary care; if anything they are underdiagnosed rather than overdiagnosed.

→ Currin L, Schmidt U, Treasure J, Jick H (2005). Time trends in eating disorder incidence. *British Journal of Psychiatry*, **186**, 132–5.

28. B ★★★   OHPsych 3rd edn → pp.304–8

BPAD (B) is slightly more common in people with higher socioeconomic status. There is a theory supporting this that suggests this condition may carry an advantage to people with it (and to unaffected family members) which would promote a rise in status, especially compared to unipolar depression and psychosis. In hypomanic or submanic states, there are periods of high industry, ideas, and promotion which create a rise in status.

Lower socioeconomic status is associated with all types of substance dependency, including alcohol dependency (A). While this is the case, it does not mean that anyone should be excluded from being asked about substance misuse. You may be surprised at what the upper-class older gentleman gets up to in his spare time.

There is a clear socioeconomic status gradient for panic disorder (C) and, in general, low socioeconomic status is associated with high psychiatric morbidity, disability, and poor access to healthcare. This may be because stress exposure, ongoing life events, and weaker social support are more prevalent in these lower status groups which puts them at risk of greater problems and delayed recovery.

The socioeconomic status of people with schizophrenia (D) is, on average, lower than the general population, but this is largely due to effects of the illness. Parental socioeconomic status of people with schizophrenia is the same as that of the general population.

Depression (E) is seen more in people with lower socioeconomic status and recent research has shown that current treatments for depression tend to favour those in employment and with a better level of social support. The focus is often on helping patients improve their ability to function at work and to use their access to local resources. More work is needed to consider how to address this disparity.

→ Bancroft A (2008). *Drugs, Intoxication and Society*. Polity Press, Cambridge.

→ Muntaner C, Eaton W, Miech R, O'Campo (2004). Socioeconomic position and major mental disorders. *Epidemiological Reviews*, **26**, 53–62.

29. B ★★★   OHPsych 3rd edn → pp.62–3, 199, 208

The answer is 20% (B). While it does not fit with lay ideas of schizophrenia, a proportion of people who receive this diagnosis will never have a further episode. The important message to deliver is that it is a myth that 'people with schizophrenia never get better', as 1 in 4–5 people with schizophrenia recover completely and another 3 out of 5 will be helped or get better with treatment.

As the woman has experienced more than one month of FRS, the ICD-10 diagnosis is schizophrenia. This is an illness where there is likely to be relapse, so a 0% (A) chance of relapse is incorrect. On the other hand, this does not mean that chronic schizophrenia is the norm. Only about 7% of people show total non-response to antipsychotic medication—resulting in a diagnosis of 'treatment-resistant schizophrenia' and different management.

Forty percent (C) is the approximate risk of developing schizophrenia if both parents have a diagnosis of schizophrenia—beware of rote learning associated facts/disorders as assessors will often use these as distractors to catch out those who don't read the question properly.

Sixty percent (D) is not the correct answer regarding psychotic episodes. For a severe depressive episode, 60% is a good estimate for the likely reoccurrence within 20 years of depression following any single depressive episode.

While 80% (E) is not an accurate answer regarding psychosis, 80% of people who have received psychiatric care for an episode of severe depression will have at least one more episode in their lifetime, with a median of four episodes.

→ RCPsych information on schizophrenia: http://www.rcpsych.ac.uk/expertadvice/problemsdisorders/schizophrenia.aspx.

30. D ★★★   OHPsych 3rd edn → p.544

The precontemplative phase (D) refers to when patients are not ready to change and not considering behaviour change at all. This patient is not concerned by her cannabis smoking and so presumably is not thinking about stopping or making any future plans about this.

The action phase of the cycle (A) occurs when a patient is actively involved in modifying or stopping the health behaviour of concern. In this case this would be the stage where this woman had stopped smoking cannabis.

The contemplative phase (B) is when a patient is thinking about making a behaviour change but not planning to do so imminently. In this case this may involve the woman considering the pros and cons of stopping smoking cannabis and considering her options and best outcomes.

The maintenance phase (C) is the 'staying on track' phase of the change cycle, where the change has successfully be made and the focus is on maintaining this and not relapsing.

The preparation phase (E) occurs just before the action phase, where a patient is actively planning an imminent change, usually within one month or so. They may have set a date for the behaviour change and planned the next stages in order to maximize their chances of success. In this case this may involve setting a quit date, telling friends and family about her plans, and thinking about ways to distract herself if she feels an urge to smoke cannabis once she has actually quit.

→ Prochaska JO, DiClemente CC (1984). *The Transtheoretical Approach: Towards a Systematic Eclectic Framework*. Dow Jones Irwin, Homewood, Illinois.

31. E ★★★   OHPsych 3rd edn → pp.1004–7

Suggesting that she take time off should be the first step (E). If she is willing to take time off, and continue with the treatment she is receiving, having a mental illness is no different to any other illness that doctors may experience. By taking time off she will be dealt with and offered support by her GP and the hospital occupational health department. As stated above, there are circumstances where you may need to involve her consultant and/or the GMC, especially around insight and willingness to accept treatment.

There is no suggestion that there is a probity issue at this point. If she refused to take time off and get treatment, or there had been a direct impact on patient care, then the GMC would need to become involved (A).

There is no evidence that the situation warrants police intervention at this point (B). As with the NHS, there needs to be a pragmatic approach to involving another agency, as too many needless referrals mean that urgent issues can be missed or urgent cases slowed.

Encouraging her to speak to her consultant would be important, but if she was willing to take a period of leave for treatment, then normal occupational health policies would be followed and you would not need to inform her consultant (C).

Offering to prescribe her risperidone is not the answer (D). Prescribing her medication would be inappropriate and go against the GMC guidelines regarding good practice in prescribing. While it is easier to spot the 'wrong answer' in these SBAs, in real life people get drawn into difficult situations trying to help our friends and colleagues, so it is important to be aware of our own behaviours.

→ GMC—Good practice in prescribing and managing medicines and devices: http://www.gmc-uk.org/Prescribing_guidance.pdf_52548623.pdf.

→ GMC—Good Medical Practice:

http://www.gmc-uk.org/guidance/good_medical_practice.asp.

→ Psychiatrist's account of her own episodes of psychotic depression: http://www.bmj.com/content/345/bmj.e6994.

32. D ★★★   OHPsych 3rd edn → pp.358, 366, 370, 372, 376

Panic disorder (D) is the only anxiety condition that is reported in equal numbers by men and women. Part of the difference between the sexes is due to health behaviour: women are more likely to report mild anxiety and depressive symptoms, but this difference is lost with more severe symptoms, e.g. having a panic attack. Another factor contributing to the apparent difference is the higher rates of substance dependency in men: alcohol dependence specifically has been associated with an underlying anxiety disorder in up to half of patients.

Women are twice as likely as men to develop generalized anxiety disorder (A).

Risk factors for mixed anxiety and depression disorder (B) include risk factors for either disorder separately. Both anxiety and depression are approximately twice as common in women as men.

OCD (C) is another anxiety disorder that has higher rates in women. OCD is characterized by intrusive thoughts that cause anxiety and distress, and is associated with repetitive behaviours that are carried out in order to reduce this distress. The practice of carrying out compulsive behaviours may temporarily reduce anxiety. However, overall these compulsions cause distress as they can be time-consuming, expensive, and embarrassing, and prevent day-to-day activities.

Specific phobias (E) are seen twice as often in women than men. The peak prevalence in early adolescence is between ages 10 and 13 years.

33. A ★★★   OHPsych 3rd edn → pp.182–5

Having a first-degree relative with schizophrenia increases the risk of developing the illness by at least tenfold (A). In twin studies of monozygotic twins raised apart, where one twin has schizophrenia, the chances of the other one (same genetic inheritance and interuterine environment, different environment after birth) having schizophrenia is 50%.

While the nature of the relationship between cannabis and the development of schizophrenia remains controversial, the Dunedin Study found that regular smoking of cannabis at age 13 was related to a two- to threefold increase in subsequent diagnoses of schizophrenia (B). Whether this is due to a chemical effect from the drug or the type of people who smoke regular cannabis at 13 years old remains to be established.

Childhood social difficulties (C) are associated with at least a fivefold increase. Although this finding is particularly susceptible to recollection bias, in prospective cohort studies non-specific childhood difficulties are associated with the development of schizophrenia. This is one of the reasons that schizophrenia is considered a neurodevelopmental disorder, with its origins prior to onset.

Immigrant status (D) is associated with up to a fivefold increase. The risk increases as the size of the immigrant community decreases in London. No clear explanation has been found for this and the specific ethnic group studied has a normal prevalence of schizophrenia in their country of origin. Interestingly the same effect is found for autism diagnosis.

There is a reported two to three times increased risk with obstetric complications (E), but at least some of this is accounted for by recollection bias (see McIntosh et al., 2002).

→ Dunedin Study: Abstract for key study: http://dunedin-study.otago.ac.nz/journals/cannabis-use-in-adolescence-and-risk-for-adult-psychosis-longitudinal-prospective-study.

→ McIntosh AM, Holmes S, Gleeson S, *et al*. (2002). Maternal recall bias, obstetric history and schizophrenia. *British Journal of Psychiatry*, **181**, 520–5.

34. D ★★★★ OHPsych 3rd edn → pp.494–7

The answer is psychopathy (D). This is not a PD. It is defined by a high score on the Psychopathy Checklist (Revised). While most people with psychopathy will meet the criteria for antisocial PD, the converse is not true.

Anankastic PD (A) is characterized by feelings of doubt, perfectionism, excessive conscientiousness, checking and preoccupation with details, stubbornness, caution, and rigidity. There may be insistent and unwelcome thoughts or impulses that do not attain the severity of an OCD.

Antisocial PD (B) is characterized by disregard for social obligations and callous unconcern for the feelings of others. There is gross disparity between behaviour and the prevailing social norms. Behaviour is not readily modifiable by adverse experience, including punishment. There is a low tolerance to frustration and a low threshold for discharge of aggression, including violence; there is a tendency to blame others, or to offer plausible rationalizations for the behaviour, bringing the patient into conflict with society.

Paranoid PD (C) is characterized by excessive sensitivity to setbacks; unforgiveness of insults; suspiciousness and a tendency to distort experience by misconstruing the neutral or friendly actions of others as hostile or contemptuous; recurrent suspicions, without justification, regarding the sexual fidelity of the spouse or sexual partner; and a combative and tenacious sense of personal rights. There may be excessive self-importance, and there is often excessive self-reference.

Schizoid PD (E) is characterized by withdrawal from affectional, social, and other contacts with preference for fantasy, solitary activities, and introspection. There is a limited capacity to express feelings and to experience pleasure.

→ ICD-10:. http://apps.who.int/classifications/icd10/browse/2010/en#/F60-F69.

35. B ★★★★ OHPsych 3rd edn → pp.9, 492–3

PDs are categories (B), defined by a number of specific descriptors. These are separate, or in some cases overlapping, categories which have a high inter-rater reliability and allow for common diagnostic criteria to be described and used. This can also be called a 'type' approach, which is a subdivision of the nomothetic approach.

Alienist (A) is the name used to describe doctors working in asylums in the Victorian era. It still infrequently appears as another name for a psychiatrist; for example, in the 1947 film *Miracle on 34th Street*, a man called Kris Kringle claims he is Santa Claus and is put on trial. In the film, several newspaper articles call the psychiatrists who examine him 'alienists'.

The dimensional approach (C) is also known as a 'trait' approach, of which IQ is the best known example of a dimensional scale. Here symptoms or any factor can be represented as numerical values on a continuum or scale, not a discrete category. Diagnosis then changes to a decision of the degree to which a particular factor is present, rather than the presence/absence of a symptom.

The ideothetic approach to personality (D) emphasizes the differences between people. It looks at what distinguishes a symptom, disorder, or condition from a similar disorder, rather than what makes up the disorder itself.

The nomothetic approach (E) looks for similarities between people. This is described as an approach to personality where people are understood in relation to societal normal values, not by their own individual uniqueness. It is the basis on which many occupational personality tests, for example the Myers–Briggs type, are based. Both categorical and divisional are subdivisions of this approach.

→ Trull TJ, Durrett CA (2005). Categorical and dimensional models of personality disorder. *Annual Review of Clinical Psychology*, **1**, 355–80.

Extended Matching Questions

1. G ★

Histrionic PD is characterized by exhibitionist, attention seeking, and overly dramatic behaviour with seductive dressing and sensitivity to others. This type of PD can often be confused with emotionally unstable PDs which are characterized by problems associated with having an unclear identity, unpredictable affect, threats or acts of self-harm, impulsivity, and intense and unstable relationships. Borderline subtypes tend to turn harm inwards (to themselves) and impulsive subtypes turn their harm outwards (on to others) where histrionic PDs do not self-harm (although they may threaten to do so for effect).

2. D ★

Dissocial PD is characterized by problems associated with having a callous lack of concern for others, irresponsibility, aggression, and an inability to keep enduring relationships. There is usually evidence of childhood conduct disorder. It can be mistaken for schizoid PD due to the unemotional nature. Dissocial PD is often accompanied by drug and alcohol problems and forensic (police) services.

3. J ★

Schizoid PD is characterized by problems associated with being emotionally cold, secretive, and (sexually) apathetic. There is an overlap with Asperger's syndrome (high functioning ASD) and the obsessive collecting and order seen in anankastic PD.

4. A ★

Anankastic PD is characterized by problems associated with having excessive doubts, caution, and perfectionist rigidity. There may be other reasons that the person may be unable to focus, for example schizophrenia (paranoid thoughts), OCD (obsessive thoughts), or disengagement with psychiatric services.

5. C ★

Dependent PD is characterized by problems associated with an excessive need for being cared for, helplessness, and submissive traits. Often it forms part of an intense relationship of dominant/submissive personalities. There are other conditions that may present in a similar manner, for example learning disability or as a result of serious past abuse.

General feedback on 1–5: OHPsych 3rd edn → pp.490–5

→ Adshead G, Sarkar J (2012). The nature of PD. *Advances in Psychiatric Treatment*, **18**, 162–72.

→ RCPsych information on personality disorders: http://www.rcpsych.
ac.uk/expertadvice/problemsdisorders/personalitydisorder.aspx.

6. G ★★

Mirtazapine can lead to prominent side-effects of increased appetite and
sedation. Most antidepressants demonstrate similar levels of efficacy in
trials, so the choice in a given patient is determined by the side-effect
profile. In some cases, side-effects can be used to the patient's benefit,
as in this case.

7. J ★★

Having tried two antidepressants from two different classes, it would be
appropriate to trial venlafaxine. It is a serotonin–noradrenaline reuptake
inhibitor (SNRI). Trials indicate it (and possibly amitriptyline) may have
slightly greater efficacy than the other antidepressants. The choice of the
SNRI over the tricyclic amitriptyline is dictated by the cardiotoxicity of
tricyclic antidepressants (TCAs) in overdose, a risk that must be considered in anyone with severe depression.

8. A ★★

TCAs such as amitriptyline and dothiepin are cardiotoxic in overdose,
due to their anticholinergic side-effects causing marked tachycardia
and arrhythmias, and it is for this reason that their use in depression
has reduced markedly over the last 20 years. Most TCAs are highly
sedating as well. Amitriptyline in low doses is also used to treat
neuropathic pain.

9. G ★★

NICE guidance recommends combining SSRIs with mirtazapine in step
3 of the treatment of depression in adults. Combining antidepressants
must be done under the supervision of a psychiatrist.

10. H ★★

Monoamine oxidase inhibitors are the oldest group of antidepressants
and work by inhibiting the breakdown of monoamines (noradrenaline,
serotonin, dopamine) by monoamine oxidase inhibitor (MAOI). They
are rarely used, however, due to the risk of the 'cheese reaction' to certain foodstuffs containing tyramine (cheese, Chianti red wines), which is
broken down by MAO. The build- up of tyramine when MAO is inhibited
by MAOIs can cause a hypertensive crisis. Moclobemide is a reversible
MAOI, whereas tranylcypromine and the other MAOIs such as phen-
elzine are irreversible. For this reason, moclobemide is the more commonly prescribed MAOI. It should be noted, however, that venlafaxine
can also cause marked hypertension.

General feedback on 5–10: OHPsych 3rd edn → pp.266–81

→ NICE—Treatment of depression in adults: http://www.nice.org.uk/nicemedia/live/12329/45890/45890.pdf.

11. G ★★

This man has five of the agreed ICD-10 symptoms of depression (low mood, anhedonia, reduced appetite, low self-esteem, and guilt or self-blame). Patients with five or six depressive symptoms are categorized as having moderate depression. This severity classification can help guide treatment options.

12. B ★★

This woman sounds as though she is currently experiencing a depressive episode and has had these in the past. The episodes of feeling full of energy and overspending are suggestive of mania or hypomania (without psychotic symptoms). Therefore she is likely to have a diagnosis of BPAD.

13. J ★★

This man has physical signs suggestive of liver disease (palmar erythema and spider naevi). Together with his occupational risk factor, it is likely that his mood symptoms are related to harmful alcohol use or alcohol dependence syndrome.

14. F ★★

This adolescent has four ICD-10 depressive symptoms (anhedonia, withdrawal, weight loss, and poor sleep). Patients with four symptoms are classified has having mild depressive disorder. She does not have dysthymia as this episode meets the criteria for a major depressive episode. Additionally in dysthymia, symptoms must be present for a longer duration: occurring on the majority of days for two years in adults, and for one year in adolescents.

15. C ★★

Cyclothymia is a chronic mood disorder where symptoms are present for most days over at least two years (one year in children and adolescents). Patients experience periods of low moods alternating with high moods, but their symptoms do not meet criteria for depressive episodes or hypomanic or manic episodes. Social, occupational, or other important areas of functioning must be affected by these mood variations for this to be classified as cyclothymia. Some clinicians believe that cyclothymia is actually a manifestation of borderline PD.

General feedback on 11–15: OHPsych 3rd edn → pp.50–1, 53, 264, 312

→ RCPsych information on bipolar disorder: http://www.rcpsych.ac.uk/healthadvice/problemsdisorders/bipolardisorder.aspx.

Chapter 5

Emergency department psychiatry

Amber Fossey

All doctors working in the ED will regularly meet patients with acute mental health problems. Five percent of total ED attendees are attributable to mental disorder. With nationwide ED attendances averaging 400 000 per week during November to April 2013, the trend shows a growing pressure on emergency services. However, these figures represent just the tip of the true burden of acute mental illness in our communities. Stigma, the healthcare funnel, and marginalization often mean that it is the sickest who finally present to the ED.

It is also important to recognize the co-morbidity of mental illness and addictions in those seeking help for what initially appear to be physical complaints, as so often the mind and body are closely intertwined.

Most common psychiatric presentations to the ED include DSH, alcohol and substance misuse, delirium, acute psychosis, factitious disorders, medically unexplained symptoms (MUS), and acute stress reactions (such as to trauma).

DSH is common but under-recognized. A quarter of people who die by suicide attended the ED in the preceding year. All patients in the ED presenting with self-harm should have a detailed psychosocial assessment.

Alcohol is responsible for 10% of all ED attendances. It is also an independent variable, raising the risk of DSH. Substance users are also frequent attendees, with high levels of medical morbidity and mortality. Patients with a dual diagnosis of substance use plus mental illness frequently present with multiple psychosocial problems.

Acute psychosis may be caused by a functional disorder, such as schizophrenia, but organic conditions must also be considered. Where a patient is extremely disturbed in the ED, restraint and sedation may be necessary to enable safe and adequate assessment. Security presence may also be required to minimize the risk of violence, where this has been identified.

Implications for working in the ED are that all doctors should familiarize themselves with the management of common acute psychiatric presentations. Know how to access local Trust rapid tranquillization guidelines. Read NICE guidelines for management of self-harm. Seize opportunities to screen for mental illness and social problems. Take a moment for health promotion. Refer onwards to crisis mental health services, secondary care, drug and alcohol services, or primary care counselling where appropriate—signposting patients to the plethora of community services available may reduce their risk of future crises.

Finally, good working relationships between the ED, psychiatry, and the community service (both primary and secondary care) are critical to successful treatment and aftercare. Carefully linking up primary care with crisis services and sharing information gives you greater confidence and reassurance that patients are being discharged safely and being followed up and supported by appropriate healthcare professionals.

Amber Fossey

QUESTIONS

Single Best Answers

1. A 23-year-old man has acute chest pain and palpitations which came on suddenly while he was shopping. He is sweaty and feels as though he is dying. His ECG and physical examination were normal and systemic enquiry revealed no other significant symptoms. Which is the *single* most likely diagnosis? ★

A Asthma

B Delusional disorder

C Depression

D Hyperthyroidism

E Panic attack

2. A 55-year-old woman with BPAD has a seizure. She has never fit- ted before. Her husband reports she had a three-day history of tremor, nausea, vomiting, muscle twitches, and bloody diarrhoea before they boarded their flight home from a holiday in Egypt. Which is the *single* most likely cause? ★

A Acute confusional state secondary to acute infection

B Lithium toxicity

C Pulmonary embolus

D Thyrotoxicosis

E Traveller's diarrhoea

3. A 48-year-old man has neglected himself to the extent he requires IV fluids to manage his dehydration. In the past, he has been given a diagnosis of schizoaffective disorder although he refused to accept this. He clearly states that any medication he is given would be useless as he is not mentally unwell. The assessing doctor is unsure of which MSE subheading to document these beliefs under. Which is the *single* most appropriate subheading to use? ★

A Insight

B Mood

C Perception

D Speech

E Thought

4. A 19-year-old woman refuses referral to plastic surgery for repair of lacerated tendons in her wrist due to DSH. The ED consultant on duty asks for an assessment of her ability to make this decision. Which is the *single* most appropriate legal framework to use? ★

A Common law

B Deprivation of Liberty Safeguards

C Mental Capacity Act

D Mental Health Act

E MMSE®-2™

5. A 68-year-old woman was admitted 24 hours earlier with headache, nausea, and anxiety. She now has a new tremor, is sweating, and has become agitated and rude to staff, demanding her medication. It is believed she is showing signs of drug withdrawal. Which is the *single* most likely medication responsible for this? ★

A Fluoxetine

B Levothyroxine

C Lorazepam

D Quetiapine

E Zopiclone

6. An 18-year-old woman has taken an overdose five hours ago. Blood tests reveal a serum paracetamol level above the treatment line. Which is the *single* most appropriate treatment to initiate? ★

A Activated charcoal

B Alkaline diuresis

C Gastric lavage

D IV Pabrinex®

E IV Parvolex®

7. A 40-year-old woman is treated in the ED for a fractured elbow after she ran into the road, partially dressed, and was hit by a cyclist. In the ED she is observed shouting obscenities and pacing about. She says she is a member of the Royal family and the newspapers will hear about her awful mistreatment. MSE shows racing thoughts, pressure of speech, and euphoric mood without disorientation. Which is the *single* most likely diagnosis? ★

A Delirium

B Drug intoxication

C Hypomania

D Mania

E Schizophrenia

8. A 51-year-old man is unwell on day two of an attempted home detox from alcohol. He is brought to the ED by his partner who is seeking help. A diagnosis of delirium tremens is suspected. Which *single* feature is most suggestive of this diagnosis? ★

A Clouding of consciousness

B Jaundice

C Suicidal thoughts

D Sweating

E Tremor

9. A 21-year-old man, whose girlfriend is in resus following a severe RTC, is 'hysterical' in the ED. At assessment, he appears dazed and detached. Which is the *single* most likely diagnosis? ★

A Abnormal grief

B Acute stress reaction

C Adjustment disorder

D Alcohol intoxication

E PTSD

10. A 47-year-old man drank antifreeze to try to end his life. He has reduced eye contact and moves quite slowly. His facial expression is flat and there are tears in his eyes. He hangs his head rather than looks up. Which is the *single* most appropriate section of the MSE to record these findings? ★

A Appearance

B Behaviour

C Cognition

D Mood

E Thought

11. A 26-year-old woman tried to remove an electronic bug from under her skin and has a deep forearm wound requiring suturing. She is, however, very agitated, pacing, and aggressive to treating staff who are unable to finish the job. It is decided that rapid tranquillization is appropriate in this case. Which is the *single* most appropriate medication to use initially? ★★

A Diazepam 10–20 mg IM

B Diazepam 10–20 mg PO

C Lorazepam 1–2 mg IM

D Lorazepam 1–2 mg PO

E Olanzapine 10–20 mg IM

12. A 46-year-old woman has a GCS score of 10/15. Ambulance staff report that they found several empty diazepam packets on her kitchen table, prescribed by her GP due to difficulty sleeping triggered by a difficult marital breakdown. Which is the *single* most appropriate medication to administer initially? ★★

A Adrenaline (epinephrine)

B Flumazenil

C N-acetylcysteine

D Naloxone

E Naltrexone

13. A 29-year-old man has had spasms in his neck and rolling of his tongue for the last day. He started taking haloperidol 10 mg once daily one week ago. Which is the *single* most appropriate description of this common side-effect? ★★

A Acute dystonia

B Akathisia

C Tardive dyskinesia

D Tics

E Parkinsonism

14. A 39-year-old man was found wandering in the road. No information was available regarding his identity and he remains mute to questioning, staring fixedly ahead. He is unkempt but not physically unwell, although his limbs are able to be passively moved into awkward postures, which he maintains for prolonged periods. Which is the *single* most likely diagnosis? ★★

A Catatonia

B Cerebrovascular event

C Depression

D Head injury

E Schizophrenia

15. A 30-year-old woman comes to the ED with palpitations and an associated tension headache. Her ECG is normal. A full history reveals that she has been worrying almost daily for several months for no apparent reason and with no subjective precipitators. She feels constantly nervous and jumpy. She has no other symptoms. Which is the *single* most likely diagnosis? ★★

A Acute stress disorder

B Generalized anxiety disorder

C Panic disorder

D Phaeochromocytoma

E Thyrotoxicosis

16. A 46-year-old man, with known alcohol dependency, is agitated and aggressive in the ED. He has a provisional diagnosis of delirium tremens. Which is the *single* most appropriate way to manage his behaviour? ★★

A Leave him to calm in a self-contained, darkened room

B Supervise him with two visible security guards present

C Treat him in a quiet, well-lit side room

D Treat him in an open bay close to the nursing station

E Use control and restraint techniques by trained staff

17. A 25-year-old man seeks protection in the ED from the 'shadow men' following him. He is hot, tachycardic, and sweaty. He admits indulging in a three-day drug binge at a festival. Which *single* drug is most likely to have caused these symptoms? ★★

A Amphetamines

B Cannabis

C Cocaine

D Ketamine

E Mushrooms

18. A 46-year-old man with alcohol dependence presents with confusion. Neurological examination reveals nystagmus and opthalmoplegia. Which is the *single* most likely other finding in this case? ★★

A Ascites

B Asterixis

C Ataxia

D Jaundice

E Pyrexia

19. A 44-year-old ex-paramedic has had severe, acute abdominal pain for the last few days. He appears agitated and crying, demanding strong painkillers and referral to surgeons. He has several old scars which appear in keeping with previously performed laparotomies. When asked he says these were performed at other hospitals. Which is the *single* most likely diagnosis? ★★★

A Depression with psychotic features

B Dissociative fugue

C Factitious disorder

D Hysteria

E Somatization

20. A 13-year-old adolescent is brought to the ED by her parents. She has burns to her forearms. She is withdrawn and tearful and cannot explain how she got the burns. Her father answers for her, saying that she fell against a hot radiator. When her parents leave the room, she asks if she can stay in hospital so she doesn't have to go home. Which *single* factor would be most likely to raise concern of child abuse? ★★★

A Below-average educational achievement

B Cuts and bruises

C Obesity

D Inconsistent explanation for injury

E Sexual naivety

21. A 35-year-old woman is transferred from an inpatient psychiatric unit with a fever, rigid muscles, sweats, tremor, and fluctuating BP. She started a depot antipsychotic three days ago. Which is the *single* most appropriate initial blood investigation? ★★★

A Creatine kinase (CK)

B C-reactive protein (CRP)

C Magnesium

D Sodium

E Thyroid stimulating hormone (TSH)

22. A 27-year-old man has been sitting in the same position in the ED for three hours, staring fixedly ahead. He has been medically cleared. MHA assessment deemed him to be mentally disordered with suspected catatonia and he is to be admitted to a psychiatric hospital. Which *single* class of medications is the most appropriate first-line treatment? ★★★

A Anticholinergic

B Antidepressant

C Antiepileptic

D Antipsychotic

E Benzodiazepine

23. A 34-year-old man falls from a ladder, resulting in a significant head injury. He is brought to the ED and successfully managed. After an admission and recovery he is ready for discharge. Part of his discharge is a follow-up appointment with a liaison psychiatrist. He is unsure why this needs to take place. Which is the *single* most likely psychiatric sequelae he may experience? ★★★★

A Cognitive impairment

B Delirium

C Persistent depression and anxiety

D Post-traumatic epilepsy

E Psychoses

24. A 60-year-old man is examined after an attempted asphyxiation by hanging. He has a clear airway with oxygen saturations of 98% but a new foot drop. Which is the *single* most likely cause for his foot drop? ★★★★

A Airway compromise

B Anterior neck soft tissue damage

C Cervical spine fracture

D Impaired consciousness

E Post-anoxic brain injury

25. A 29-year-old woman has dizziness, headaches, nausea, and sensations in her legs which she describes as being like 'electric shocks'. She had been prescribed psychotropic medication four months ago but recently stopped taking it as she felt a lot better. She had not consulted her GP or tapered off her dosage. Which is the *single* most likely medication she was prescribed? ★★★★

A Lithium

B Paroxetine

C Propranolol

D Quetiapine

E Temazepam

Extended Matching Questions

Emergency investigations

The following clinical scenarios all present to the ED over a bank holiday weekend. Before requesting input from the Liaison Psychiatry team, each patient should be thoroughly assessed. Select the *single* most appropriate investigation for each clinical scenario. ★★

A Blood glucose

B CT scan of head

C ECG

D EEG

E GCS

F LFTs

G MMSE®-2™

H MSE

I Thyroid function tests (TFTs)

J Urine dipstick

1. A 72-year-old woman is confused, disorientated, and talking to herself. Her husband says that she hasn't been herself for a couple of days: more fractious, inattentive, and needing to go to the lavatory more than usual.

2. A 40-year-old man is known to have schizophrenia which has been unresponsive to medication. Three weeks ago he was commenced on a new medication, the name of which he can't remember, which has been slowly increased. He has felt unwell for a few days, then today developed chest pain and breathlessness.

3. A 28-year-old woman comes to the ED in tears as she feels she can't go on living. She is dishevelled and smells unwashed. She has with her an 18-month-old baby who appears healthy.

4. A 49-year-old man is brought into the ED by the police having sustained an ankle injury during arrest. He was observed to have attacked his wife. He says that he cannot remember anything about this attack. His wife says he has had three episodes this year of losing his temper and lashing out.

5. A 46-year-old mother of four asks for help as she feels she 'can't cope anymore'. She is very anxious, wringing her hands, sweating, and trembling. She describes losing weight over recent months, being up all night, having palpitations, and feeling hot all the time.

Post-partum psychiatry

For each of the following scenarios, choose the *single* most appropriate diagnosis from the list of options below. Each option may be used once, more than once, or not at all. ★★

A Baby blues

B BPAD

C Cyclothymia

D Delusional disorder

E Mixed anxiety and depressive disorder

F Post-natal depression

G Post-partum PTSD

H Psychotic depression

I Puerperal psychosis

J Schizophrenia

6. A 34-year-old woman brings her two-month-old boy to the ED with a cough. The baby appears to have a minor upper respiratory tract infection (URTI) but nothing more serious. Despite this, she is inconsolable with worry. She has felt this way for three weeks, has lost her appetite, and has had guilty thoughts that she is a bad mother.

7. A 29-year-old woman has been experiencing difficulties since the birth of her son, by emergency caesarean section eight weeks ago. She has had difficulty sleeping due to recurring nightmares and, when awake, has had sudden images of surgeons slicing open her stomach. She has been acutely sensitive to her baby's noises, checking on him every few minutes. She was very scared about coming into the ED as she felt this made her anxiety much worse.

8. A husband brings his 32-year-old wife to the ED after she told him their two-week-old boy has the devil inside him and must be killed for the good of humanity.

9. A 25-year-old woman brings her four-day-old girl to the ED with jaundice. While the baby is being examined, it is seen that the mother cries non-stop at the bedside. She says she has felt low and tired since the delivery.

10. A 28-year-old woman has had low mood, early morning waking, and poor appetite for six weeks. She has a 15-month-old daughter with her. She had a similar low episode seven years ago and was admitted to hospital four years ago with overactivity, insomnia, and a delusion that she was a member of the Swedish Royal family.

Neurological deficit

For each scenario below, choose the *single* most appropriate neurological deficit from the list of options. Each option may be used once, more than once, or not at all. Match each definition with the correct term. ★★★

A Anosognosia

B Aphasia

C Astasia-abasia

D Asterognosia

E Bradyphrenia

F Dysarthria

G Finger agnosia

H Hemiasomatognosia

I Prosopagnosia

J Simultagnosia

11. A 64-year-old woman has a stroke which left her with right-sided weakness. She says that she feels normal despite this weakness being demonstrated by the doctor examining her. This has resulted in her dropping a heavy tin on her foot.

12. A 34-year-old man is waiting for the results of an emergency chest X-ray. He tells the nurse that people keep stealing and replacing his belongings while he isn't paying attention. He has on his table a phone, wallet, and watch and can only see the object he is focused on, believing the others have disappeared. As soon as his attention is refocused on another object, he can see it clearly but believes the other objects are now gone.

13. A 27-year-old man has difficulty explaining why he has come to the ED. He says disjointed words such as 'Emily' (his wife's name)...'hospital...scared...scared...no'. Even trying to write down his problem results in the same halting pattern.

14. A 71-year-old man fell, damaging his ankle, and was brought to the ED. His wife arrives to collect him but he says that he doesn't know who the woman is. When she steps outside with the ED doctor, he hears her talking and says 'That's my wife's voice'.

15. A 24-year-old man has a seizure and is taken to the ED. He is found to have a non-dominant hemispherical lesion. Whilst being assessed he claims to be unable to recognize an object, such as his keys, when he holds them in his hand with his eyes shut.

ANSWERS

Single Best Answers

1. E ★   OHPsych 3rd edn → pp.358–9

Panic attack (E) is the correct answer. A panic attack is a period of intense fear characterized by clusters of symptoms which include palpitations, sweating, trembling, shortness of breath, feeling of choking, chest pain, nausea, dizziness, derealization, and a fear of losing control or dying. They develop rapidly, peak in intensity around ten minutes, and rarely last more than an hour. Community services show co-morbidity with agoraphobia of 30–50%. In this case, the panic attack seems to have been precipitated by social anxiety in a crowded public place. Sufferers may seek help from medical services fearing acute physical illness, such as a heart attack.

Asthma (A) would likely be revealed by a patient's previous medical history and wheeze on respiratory examination.

Delusional disorder (B) is an uncommon condition where patients present with circumscribed symptoms of non-bizarre delusions, but with an absence of perceptual or mood disorder. They rarely present directly to psychiatrists, more often being seen by other physicians due to somatic complaints, or lawyers and police due to paranoid ideas. Panic attacks have an anxiety basis rather than a delusional construct.

Anxiety with panic attacks may be associated with depression (C), but the features in this case are not of core depressive symptoms.

Hyperthyroidism (D) can cause restlessness, nervousness, tremor, and sweating, but the context here is of acute symptoms triggered by a social context.

→ NHS Choices—panic disorder: http://www.nhs.uk/conditions/panic-disorder/pages/introduction.aspx.

2. B ★   OHPsych 3rd edn → pp.338–40

Lithium (B) is the most likely cause. Lithium is a mood-stabilizing drug used in BPAD, though also in cases of treatment-resistant depression or psychotic illness with a strong affective component. Lithium has a narrow therapeutic index. Toxicity may be precipitated by inadequate hydration and salt intake. Early signs of toxicity include marked tremor, anorexia, nausea, vomiting, and diarrhoea (sometimes bloody), with associated dehydration and lethargy. As lithium levels rise, severe neurological complications such as hypertonicity and myoclonic jerks can occur. This may progress to ataxia, delirium, cardiac arrhythmias, seizures, coma, and death. Olanzapine is an antipsychotic medication with mood-stabilizing properties that may be prescribed in BPAD. It can cause metabolic syndrome and sedation, but high serum levels are not associated with a toxic syndrome akin to lithium.

Acute confusional state secondary to acute infection (A) is unlikely in this case as it doesn't fit the clinical picture. It includes severe confusion and disorientation, developing with relatively rapid onset and fluctuating in intensity. It is more usual in elderly patients.

Recent air travel may be a risk factor for pulmonary embolus (C), but the symptoms described here are not classical for thromboses.

Thyrotoxicosis (D) is characterized by signs of sympathetic overactivity such as tremor, tachycardia, and sweating producing weight loss, fatigue, and heat intolerance. Lithium therapy can cause hypothyroidism but not hyperthyroidism.

Traveller's diarrhoea (E) could be suspected in a patient with diarrhoea returning from abroad, but seizures and muscle twitches would be unlikely.

→ Patient.co.uk—lithium factsheet: http://www.patient.co.uk/doctor/lithium-pro.

3. A ★   OHPsych 3rd edn → pp.44–5

Insight (A) is the correct answer. Insight assesses the patient's experience of illness and their views towards treatment. This includes whether they will accept medical advice and treatment.

Mood (B) entails a subjective and objective assessment of mood states and associated symptomatology.

Perception (C) includes hallucinations, illusions, derealization, and depersonalization.

Speech (D) covers volume, rate, and tone, plus quantity and fluency.

Thought (E) involves assessment for formal thought disorder as well as delusions and overvalued ideas.

→ http://www.trickcyclists.co.uk/osces_MSE.htm.

4. C ★   OHPsych 3rd edn → pp.794–5, 880–1

The answer is the Mental Capacity Act (C). The issue of treating patients without consent arises frequently in a psychiatric context. Capacity is a legal concept meaning the ability to enter into valid contracts. It is gained on adulthood and presumed to be present unless permanently or temporarily lost. Doctors may be called on to give an assessment of capacity in order to decide on the ability of a patient to give informed consent. The questions to ask are only relevant to the decision required of them in that case. It asks does the patient have the ability to: (1) make a decision, (2) understand the information relevant to the decision, (3) retain memory of the decision, and (4) communicate the decision.

Common law (A) may allow for emergency treatment to preserve life where it is not possible to obtain consent. It does not apply to assessment of a conscious patient's ability to give consent, as is being questioned here.

Deprivation of Liberty Safeguards (B) are designed to protect the inter-ests of vulnerable service users such as those with dementia or learning disability and to ensure people can be given the care they need in the least restrictive regimes.

The Mental Health Act 1983 (amended 2007) applies to compulsory detention and treatment of people with mental disorder and is not used to assess capacity (D).

MMSE®-2™ (E) is a brief 30-point questionnaire test that is used to screen for cognitive impairment. It is commonly used in medicine to screen for dementia but does not assess capacity.

→ Mental Capacity Act: http://www.justice.gov.uk/protecting-the-vulnerable/mental-capacity-act.

5. C ★   OHPsych 3rd edn → p.600

The constellation of symptoms above are classic for benzodiazepine with-drawal. Lorazepam (C) is one of the shortest-acting benzodiazepines. If taken regularly and for a long enough period to develop dependence, withdrawal symptoms would be expected to be seen if suddenly stopped.

Fluoxetine (A) is the SSRI antidepressant with the longest half-life, so it would not cause withdrawal effects for many days.

Levothyroxine (B) is a treatment for hypothyroidism that does not have side-effects of tolerance or dependence.

Quietiapine (D) is an atypical antipsychotic, which neither is generally addictive nor causes withdrawal symptoms.

Zopiclone (E) is a hypnotic used for night sedation. If relied on for sleep initiation for longer than two weeks, rebound insomnia may occur.

6. E ★   OHPsych 3rd edn → p.986

The most appropriate treatment is IV Parvolex® (E). Plasma paracetamol concentrations should be measured in all conscious patients with a history of paracetamol overdose, or suspected paracetamol overdose, as recom-mended by TOXBASE. They should also be taken in patients with a pre-sentation consistent with opioid poisoning, and in unconscious patients with a history of collapse where drug overdose is a possible diagnosis. Plasma paracetamol levels should be measured for risk assessment no earlier than four hours and no later than 15 hours after ingestion, as results are not reliable outside this time period. IV acetylcysteine (Parvolex®) should be considered as the treatment of choice for paracetamol overdose.

When a person who has self-poisoned is in the ED within one hour of inges-tion and is fully conscious and able to protect his or her own airway, ED staff should consider offering activated charcoal (A) at the earliest opportunity. In this scenario the patient has presented too late for this to be an option.

Forced alkaline diuresis (B) is indicated in the treatment of moderate salicylate poisoning only. It should not be used if the patient is in shock, has heart failure, or has impaired renal function.

NICE guidelines state that gastric lavage (C) should not be used in the management of self-poisoning unless specifically recommended by TOXBASE or following consultation with the National Poisons Information Service.

Pabrinex® (D) is the brand name for a high-potency injection containing the water-soluble vitamins C (ascorbic acid), B_1 (thiamine), B_2 (riboflavin), B_3 (nicotinamide), and B_6 (pyridoxine). It is administered during alcohol withdrawal to prevent Wernicke's encephalitis.

→ NICE Clinical Guideline 16—Self-harm: http://www.nice.org.uk/nicemedia/live/10946/29421/29421.pdf.

7. D ★   OHPsych 3rd edn → pp.306–7

The constellation of symptoms in this case strongly suggests mania (D). For diagnosis, symptoms should have been present for at least one week. Classic symptoms include elevated mood, increased energy (which may manifest as pressured speech and racing thoughts), grandiosity, distractibility, risky behaviour, and agitation. Marked disruption of occupational and social functioning is usually seen. Psychotic symptoms may or may not occur, and are usually mood congruent.

Delirium (A) is an acute confusional state characterized by fluctuant mental state, altered level of consciousness, and emotional, psychomotor, and cognitive disturbance. It has an organic origin. It would be unlikely for an elbow injury, as in the case above, to precipitate delirium, unless later complicated, for example by infection. There has been no suggestion of a head injury.

There is no indication from the case above that the patient is intoxicated with drugs or alcohol (B). Depending on substance used, presentations from drug intoxication and withdrawal vary widely.

Hypomania (C) differs from mania in that symptoms are present to a lesser degree and do not significantly disrupt work or social life. They must be present for at least four days. Psychotic symptoms are excluded.

A patient with schizophrenia (E) may present with mood-congruent delusions, but primarily symptoms are of perceptual disturbance and delusions. If mood swings are a prominent and persistent feature the patient may be considered to have schizoaffective disorder, a disorder somewhere on the continuum between BPAD and psychotic illness.

8. A ★   OHPsych 3rd edn → pp.558–9

Delirium tremens is an acute confusional state secondary to alcohol withdrawal and is an emergency medical condition requiring inpatient care. In addition to the features of uncomplicated alcohol withdrawal there is clouding of consciousness (A), disorientation, retrograde amnesia, psychomotor agitation, hallucinations, and marked fluctuations. It occurs in 5% of those with alcohol withdrawal, with a peak incidence at 48 hours. It has a mortality rate of 5–10%.

Jaundice (B) is a feature of decompensated liver disease, which may be seen as a complication of chronic alcohol dependence in a case of withdrawal, but is not pathognomic of withdrawal itself.

Suicidal thoughts (C) may be present in any altered mental state associated with affective symptoms, though symptoms of fear and paranoia with visual, tactile, and auditory hallucinations tend to be associated with delirium tremens.

Sweating (D) is a feature of uncomplicated alcohol withdrawal.

Coarse tremor (E) is a feature of uncomplicated alcohol withdrawal. These tremors are usually seen as relatively slow movements which involve larger muscle groups.

9. B ★　　　OHPsych 3rd edn → p.382

Acute stress reaction (B) is a response within one hour to exceptional stress. It is a transient disorder lasting hours or days. Symptoms may be mixed or changeable, but include initial daze, anger, despair, disorientation, aggression, and hopelessness.

Abnormal grief (A) may occur after a bereavement and refers to a very intense, prolonged, delayed, or absent grief reaction, where symptoms outside the normal range are seen.

Adjustment disorder (C) is a brief depressive reaction occurring within one month of a psychosocial stressor and lasting less than six months.

There is no indication in the scenario that the patient is intoxicated (D). He should not presume to be so unless signs indicate this is a factor to take into consideration.

PTSD (E) symptoms arise within six months of the traumatic event and are characterized by involuntary re-experiencing of the event, with hyperarousal, avoidance, and emotional numbing.

→ Bryant RA (2006). Acute stress disorder. *Psychiatry*, **5** (7), 238–9.

10. B ★　　　OHPsych 3rd edn → pp.44–5

Behaviour (B) is the correct section to document these observations. It is documented second, after describing appearance. This will include appropriateness of behaviour, level of motor activity, eye contact, rapport, abnormal posture, aggression, or tearfulness.

The greater part of the MSE consists of empathic questioning about the patient's internal experiences. Nonetheless, important information regarding mental state can be obtained from careful observation of the patient's appearance (A), behaviour, and manner. The patient's physical appearance should be documented first. This will include racial origin, comparison of biological age with chronological age, manner of dress, level of cleanliness, general physical condition, and abnormal involuntary movements.

Cognition (C) broadly covers the patient's level of consciousness, clarity of thought, orientation, memory, and intellect. This may be briefly screened using a 10-item abbreviated mental test or 30-point MMSE®-2™.

Mood (D) should entail a subjective account and objective assessment. Mood evaluation includes quality, range, congruence, and appropriateness of the mood state. Anxiety and panic should be asked about here, plus obsessions and compulsions. Suicidal ideation or intent should also be quantified.

Under thought (E), both content and form should be explored. Content describes the meaning of beliefs, perception, and memory, as felt by the patient. Form describes the structure and process of thought; for example racing thoughts. Speech is the only objective representation of thought form, but it may also be elicited by careful questioning of the patient's subjective experience.

11. D ★★   OHPsych 3rd edn → pp.990–1

Local protocols for rapid tranquillization and control and restraint should be followed. However, it is important to use the least restrictive measure and work with the patient as far as possible to reduce risk of harm to patient and others. Oral (PO) medication should be offered first line, with escalation to IM medication only where oral medication has failed, been refused, or is not indicated.

Oral lorazepam 1–2 mg (D) should be offered first line in this case. IV medication should only be used in exceptional circumstances where immediate tranquillization is necessary. Thus diazepam 10–20 mg IM (A) is not the correct answer.

Diazepam 10–20 mg PO (B) is not recommended for rapid tranquillization because of its slower onset of action and longer duration compared with shorter-acting benzodiazepines.

Lorazepam is the benzodiazepine of choice for rapid tranquillization, 1–2 mg both for PO and IM dosing (C). This may be combined with haloperidol if psychosis is present.

Olanzapine IM (E) may be considered second line for moderate disturbance, but must not be given within one hour of IM lorazepam.

12. B ★★   OHPsych 3rd edn → pp.68–9

Flumazenil (B) is a gamma-aminobutyric acid (GABA) antagonist, available for injection only, which can be used as an antidote in the treatment of benzodiazepine overdoses. Long-acting benzodiazepines such as diazepam may require repeated administration of flumazenil due to its short half-life. Diazepam is a benzodiazepine medication commonly used for short-term relief of anxiety and sleeping problems.

Adrenaline (A) has various uses in emergency medicine, but reversal of benzodiazepine overdose is not one of them. Many generic drug names have been changed following recommended International Non-Proprietary Name (rINN) rules. However, adrenaline (epinephrine) and noradrenaline (norepinephrine) will continue to be called by both names because it was believed to be too risky given their widespread use in emergency medicine.

N-acetylcysteine (C) is used in the management of paracetamol overdose.

Naloxone (D) is an opioid inverse agonist drug, used to counter the effects of opiate overdose.

Naltrexone (E) is an opioid receptor antagonist used primarily in the management of alcohol dependence and opioid dependence.

→ British National Formulary—emergency treatment of poisoning: www.bnf.org.

→ www.toxbase.org.

13. **A** ★★   OHPsych 3rd edn → pp.954–5

Acute dystonia (A) is the most appropriate description. This is a reaction following exposure to antipsychotic medication with sustained, often painful muscular spasms. Most frequent are neck dystonias, followed by tongue and jaw. Incidence is 3–10% of patients exposed to antipsychotics (up to 30% with high-potency drugs). Younger age group, males, and high-potency antipsychotics confer higher risk. Ninety percent of the onset of symptoms occurs within the first five days of exposure.

Akathisia (B) is a subjective feeling of inner restlessness and objective psychomotor agitation (such as pacing) associated with antipsychotic medication.

Tardive dyskinesia (C) is characterized by involuntary, repetitive, and purposeless movements occurring with long-term antipsychotic exposure of months to years.

A tic (D) is a sudden, repetitive, non-rhythmic motor movement or vocalization involving discrete muscle groups. Tics are not a common side-effect of antipsychotic medication.

Parkinsonism (E) is a frequent adverse effect in around 20% of patients treated with antipsychotic medication. Parkinson's disease is a progressive neurological condition not associated with antipsychotic medication per se.

→ YouTube video of acute dystonia: http://www.youtube.com/watch?v=Gjiy1rDZpp8.

14. **A** ★★   OHPsych 3rd edn → pp.992–3

The most likely diagnosis is catatonia (A). Characteristic signs of catatonia are mutism, posturing, negativism, staring, rigidity, and echopraxia or echolalia. Bizarre motor presentations include waxy flexibility (where limbs are able to be passively moved into awkward postures which are maintained for prolonged periods). Catatonia has multifactorial aetiologies but is an important condition to recognize, as excited forms left untreated can become lethal.

A differential diagnosis would be a cerebrovascular event (B) as mutism can be associated with focal neurological signs. A differentiating feature would be that a stroke patient will often try to communicate by other means.

Catatonia is more often associated with mania (it accounts for up to 50% of cases). When associated with a mood state, it is generally referred to as a manic or depressive stupor (C).

Head injury (D) may be a cause of delirium, but you may expect other focal neurological signs or a clear point of injury such a bruise or scar.

Ten to fifteen percent of cases of catatonia occur in patients with schizophrenia (E). However, the signs presented here are diagnostic of catatonia and are not pathognomic of schizophrenia as a disorder.

15. B ★★   OHPsych 3rd edn → pp.372–4

The most likely diagnosis is generalized anxiety disorder (B). This has been described by NICE as 'a very common but under-recognized condition characterized by endless worrying, which results in substantial disability for many sufferers, affecting their capacity to work and to live fulfilled and meaningful lives'. Its symptoms are hard to define as they are a near-constant free-floating anxiety about everything with some somatic symptoms but with no clear causative or alleviating behaviours. People with generalized anxiety disorder may appear outwardly 'ordinary' but are actually managing significant worries. There is often an acute-on-chronic element to the disorder with symptoms changing over time to have more, or less, effect on activities of daily living.

Acute stress disorder (A) would arise following a significant trauma. Without this event it would be unlikely this would be the diagnosis. There is an overlap of symptoms with a generalized anxiety disorder, as both can include agitation and anxiety, or with a panic disorder: where there is autonomic arousal, tachycardia, sweating, etc. It is important to always ask about events occurring before the symptoms start and any clear precipitating factors.

Panic disorder (C), or panic attack, involves periods of acute anxiety or fear which start suddenly and can last from minutes to hours, usually peaking at about ten minutes. There are associated features of depersonalization, dizziness, and fears of losing control or dying. Many people describe them as intensely frightening and in themselves a traumatic experience. For a panic disorder to be diagnosed there should be a discrete period of anxiety, with a peak and fall, and at least four symptoms of sympathetic nervous system response: palpitations, sweating, shortness of breath, nausea, paraesthesias, dizziness, etc. In this scenario, the anxiety is more free-floating, constant, and without a start or stop.

Phaeochromocytoma (D) is a neuroendocrine tumour of the medulla of the adrenal glands where high levels of catecholamines are secreted, leading to sympathetic nervous system hyperactivity as described above. Most worryingly there is a rise in blood pressure which can be dangerous, and is poorly controlled with antihypertensive medication. It is an organic condition which should be considered when 'psychiatric' symptoms are present, as missing it can be fatal. Diagnosis is by plasma or 24-hour urinary measurements of catecholamines.

Thyrotoxicosis (E) can be confused with generalized anxiety disorder as both have increased subjective anxiety with palpitations, and headaches. However, in thyrotoxicosis there would be characteristic signs of a tremor, weight loss, and heat intolerance. These are associated with an overactive thyroid resulting in excessive concentrations of free thyroid hormones in the blood. A simple bedside test is to examine the hands; in thyrotoxicosis they are likely to be sweaty, tremulous, and warm, rather than cold and clammy in anxiety (where there is peripheral vasoconstriction). Routine TFTs would confirm the diagnosis.

→ Iacovides A, Fountoulakis KN, Grammaticos P, Ierodiakonou C (2000). Difference in symptom profile between generalized anxiety disorder and anxiety secondary to hyperthyroidism. *International Journal of Psychiatry in Medicine*, **30** (1), 71–81. → Phaeochromocytoma: BMJ 2012;344:e1042.

16. **C** ★★   OHPsych 3rd edn → pp.558–9

The most appropriate way to manage his behaviour is to treat him in a quiet, well-lit side room (C). Good lighting is important to aid orientation. It is helpful to have a board in the room with the date and place clearly stated and a working clock. It is also known that excessive noise, particularly white noise, stimulates a patient and can agitate them, hence a quiet environment is best. While this may not always be totally achievable in the busy ED it is best to aim for this environment.

Leaving him to calm in a self-contained, darkened room (A) ignores the supportive measures important in the management of delirium. A darkened room would worsen disorientation and confusion. Leaving a patient in a room to 'calm down' is dangerous and could lead to further injury or worsening physical health.

It is always important to ensure the safety of all healthcare professions, as well as other patients and the patient themselves; however, two visible security guards (B) might intimidate the patient and worsen aggression. It is also important to clarify what role the security guards think they are playing—is it to prevent an unwell patient from leaving, prevent property damage or theft, or ensure that an aggressive patient without any physical/mental health needs leaves the ED without fuss.

Excessive sensory input, as would occur in an open bay, is best avoided (D). There should not be an expectation that being 'close to nursing station' means that more attention will be placed on the patient. If there is a concern that this patient needs 1:1 observation then this should be clearly stated in the notes.

Physical restraint should be avoided (E), as least restrictive measures should always be used first. If it is necessary then it should only be delivered by an appropriate number of trained staff with a clear plan in place regarding the purpose of the restraint—for example to deliver IM medication or to move the patient to a safer location.

→ NICE Clinical Guideline 103—Delirium: http://www.nice.org.uk/nicemedia/live/13060/49908/49908.pdf.

17. **A** ★★   OHPsych 3rd edn → p.585

The answer is amphetamines (A). These are stimulant drugs used recreationally to make users feel alert and chatty, hence the street name 'speed'. Acute harmful effects include tachycardia, hyperpyrexia, and a quasi-psychotic state with visual, auditory, and tactile hallucinations. Acute amphetamine intoxication can mimic schizophrenia but needs to be differentiated; a careful history here is helpful.

Cannabis intoxication (B) can cause mild tachycardia and mild paranoia, but delusions and hallucinations would not be seen as an acute effect. Chronic cannabis use, especially from an early age, is a risk factor associated with development of schizophrenia.

Cocaine (C) is a stimulant drug causing increased energy, confidence, and euphoria. Acute harmful effects include arrhythmias, anxiety, and hypertension. Acute psychosis is not seen.

Ketamine (D) is a hallucinogenic anaesthetic used recreationally for dissociative experiences. Common acute side-effects are nausea, ataxia, and slurred speech.

Magic mushrooms (E) in small doses can cause euphoria, while large doses can cause perceptual abnormalities such as visual distortions, synaesthesia, and distorted body image. Harmful effects include nausea, vomiting, and diarrhoea.

→ http://www.talktofrank.com/drug/speed.

18. C ★★   OHPsych 3rd edn → pp.572–3

This man presents with the tetrad of symptoms seen in Wernicke's encephalopathy: acute confusional state, ataxia (C), and nystagmus and opthalmoplegia. Wernicke's encephalopathy is caused by thiamine deficiency, often from prolonged alcohol consumption. Untreated it may progress to Korsakoff psychosis, coma, and death.

Ascites (A) is a feature of decompensated liver disease. Liver disease may be associated with chronic alcohol dependence but is not a diagnostic feature of Wernicke's encephalopathy. Ascites is confirmed on physical examination. There is a visible abdominal bulge with 'shifting dullness'—a difference in percussion which shifts when the patient turns onto their side.

Asterixis (B), or liver flap, is a gross motor tremor of the hand. It is seen when the wrist is extended then bent upwards with the arm outstretched. It is caused by abnormal function of the diencephalic motor centres in the brain, which regulate the muscles involved in maintaining position. It is a feature of decompensated liver disease and can also be seen in Wilson's disease or carbon monoxide toxicity.

Jaundice (D) is often seen in hepatitis or in other liver disease, such as liver cancer, or obstruction of the biliary tract. It is present in many people with alcoholic liver disease but is not a diagnostic feature of Wernicke's encephalopathy.

Pyrexia (E) is unrelated to Wernicke's encephalopathy. It may be related to an untreated infection, such as a urinary tract infection (UTI), which in turn could lead to delirium.

→ Alzheimer's Society factsheet: What is Korsakoff's syndrome? http://www.alzheimers.org.uk/site/scripts/documents_info. php?documentID=98.

19. C ★★★ OHPsych 3rd edn → pp.814–15

The most likely diagnosis is factitious disorder (C). In this disorder patients intentionally falsify their symptoms and past history with the primary aim of obtaining medical attention. The 'wandering' subtype consists of mostly males, who move from hospital to hospital producing dramatic stories. Factitious disorder was previously known as Münchausen's. Risk factors for developing factitious disorder include working in the health-care profession, or having aspirations to do so. It is more common in men and seen in younger and middle-aged adults. Other risk factors include childhood illness, trauma, and parents with illnesses.

In depression a patient may be more likely to experience somatic symptoms of anxiety and biological symptoms such as poor sleep, low energy, and reduced appetite (A). In severe depression with psychotic features a patient may develop mood-congruent delusions, such as nihilistic ideas that their internal organs are rotting away. However, these ideas are not being driven by a desire for medical attention and would be unlikely to present like the scenario above.

Dissociative disorders (also known as conversion) occur when there is a loss of normal function which initially appears to have a physical cause but is proven to be psychological. Symptoms, however, are not produced intentionally. A fugue state (B) is a dissociative reaction to extreme stress, where the individual develops global amnesia and may wander to a distant location.

Hysteria (D) is an outdated term no longer used in modern medicine. It was replaced within the category of somatization disorders before being officially changed from 'hysterical neurosis' to conversion disorder. The name itself was assumed to be particular to women and caused by disturbances of the uterus. In the 19th century, hysteria was treated by massage of the patient's genitalia (by the physician) or by vibrators or water sprays to cause orgasm.

In somatization disorder (E) patients do not consciously produce symptoms or fabricate history. It is sometimes called Briquet's syndrome.

→http://www.mind.org.uk/help/medical_and_alternative_care/making_sense_of_coming_off_psychiatric_drugs.

20. D ★★★ OHPsych 3rd edn → pp.662–3

Important indicators of physical abuse are bruises or injuries that are either unexplained or inconsistent with the explanation given by the parents (D). Recognizing child abuse is not easy. It is not your responsibility to decide whether or not child abuse has taken place or if a child is at significant risk of harm from someone. You do, however, have both a responsibility and duty to act in order that the appropriate agencies can investigate and take any necessary action to protect a child.

Below-average academic achievement (A) would not on its own raise suspicion of abuse, although a significant change in school performance may be a sign that a child is under some form of stress.

Most children will collect cuts and bruises (B) as part of the rough-and-tumble of daily life. Injuries should always be interpreted in light of the child's medical and social history, developmental stage, and the explanation given.

The physical signs of neglect may include constant hunger, sometimes stealing food from other children, loss of weight, or being constantly underweight (rather than obesity) (C).

Changes in behaviour that can indicate sexual abuse include sexual knowledge that is beyond their age or developmental level (rather than naivety) (E).

→ NSPCC Child Protection Fact Sheet: http://www.nspcc.org.uk/inform/trainingandconsultancy/consultancy/helpandadvice/definitions_and_signs_of_child_abuse_pdf_wdf65412.pdf.

21. A ★★★ OHPsych 3rd edn → pp.956–8

The answer is CK (A). This question tests appropriate investigation for neuroleptic malignant syndrome (NMS). NMS is a rare, life-threatening, idiosyncratic reaction to antipsychotic (and other) medications characterized by fever, muscular rigidity, altered mental status, and autonomic dysfunction. High-potency antipsychotic and depot preparations are known risk factors. Raised serum CK is associated with NMS.

CRP (B) is produced by the liver. The level of CRP rises when there is inflammation throughout the body. CRP might well be raised in infection leading to delirium (altered mental state) and fever, but this is unlikely here.

Deficiency of magnesium (C) causes muscle cramps, tremors (due to increased irritability of the nervous system), and confusion. However, it is usually a chronic condition caused by poor diet, diarrhoea, or medication such as diuretics. It is unlikely to appear within three days. It can be seen within a psychiatric setting as hypomagnesaemia occurs in a third of alcoholics, and almost all delirium tremens inpatients, due to malnutrition and chronic diarrhoea.

Deficiency of sodium (D) is unlikely in this presentation but something to consider in a patient with new-onset altered mental state. Symptoms of hyponatraemia include muscle weakness, spasms, seizures, and lethargy. Symptom severity is associated with serum sodium levels: the lower the serum sodium the more prominent and serious the symptoms. Neurological symptoms typically occur only with very low levels of serum sodium (< 115 mEq/L). Here excess water entering brain cells causes them to swell, which results in encephalopathy which is life threatening.

TSH testing will reveal underlying hypothyroidism and hyperthyroidism. Although hyperthyroidism (E) will produce a tremor, sweats, and raised BP, it would not account for the rigidity or fever. As NMS (a more likely diagnosis) is life threatening, this is something that should be investigated and ruled out first.

→ Adnet P, Lestavel P, Krivosic-Horber R (2000). Neuroleptic malignant syndrome. *British Journal of Anaesthesia*, **85** (1), 129–35.

22. E ★★★   OHPsych 3rd edn → pp.992–3

Best evidence for treatment of catatonia is for benzodiazepines (E), e.g. lorazepam PO or IM. Barbiturates, though less widely used, may also be tried, as may electroconvulsive therapy (ECT). Alone or in combination, these drugs effectively relieve catatonic symptoms regardless of severity in 70–80% of cases. Any underlying medical or psychiatric disorder should also be addressed.

Anticholinergic drugs (A), such as procyclidine, are generally used within psychiatry for the relief of extrapyramidal side-effects caused by antipsychotic medication. They would not be effective for treatment of catatonia.

Antidepressants (B) generally take some weeks to reach therapeutic effect, so would not be beneficial for the acute management of a catatonic state. They may still be useful clinically if depression is an underlying cause.

Antiepileptic medications (C) are not licensed for the management of catatonia.

Antipsychotic medication (D) is not the pharmacological treatment of choice in catatonia, but may well be considered as an adjunct if the underlying illness is felt to be psychotic in nature.

23. C ★★★★   OHPsych 3rd edn → pp.260–1

Depressive illness is most common, but anxiety states are common sequelae. Persistent depression and anxiety (C) occurs in roughly 25% of head injury survivors.

Most head injury survivors who present to psychiatric services have emotional symptoms and personality changes ranging from subtle to severe. A smaller number manifest serious and lasting cognitive sequelae, such as apathy, disinhibition, and amnesia. Cognitive impairment (A) is more likely after closed head injuries, with post-traumatic amnesia lasting more than 24 hours.

Acute post-traumatic delirium (B) may follow severe head injury as the patient regains consciousness. Often this is in the context of forced alcohol withdrawal or due to the unrecognized environment and situation causing acute confusion.

Post-traumatic epilepsy (D) occurs in 5% of closed and 30% of open head injuries. Preventative anti-epileptics, given before symptoms are seen, do not prevent the development of post-traumatic epilepsy after head injury.

Psychoses (E) are not the most likely psychiatric sequelae he experienced. There is an increased risk of schizophrenia post head injury;

2.5% develop the disorder. The risk of developing schizophrenia has not been shown to increase in more severe brain injuries, which suggests that trauma location has more effect than total damage. There is also a question of whether sustaining a head injury brings people into hospital, resulting in a full assessment where previously undiagnosed psychotic illness is found, or if a new worsening psychotic illness causes risky behaviours which can result in head injuries (or both).

→ Kanner A (ed.) (2012). *Depression in Neurologic Disorders: Diagnosis and Management.* Wiley-Blackwell, Oxford.

24. C ★★★★ OHPsych 3rd edn → p.987

Cervical spine fractures (C) should be considered if there is a possibility of foot drop or evidence of focal neurological deficit.

Airway compromise is not the right answer (A). Most victims of attempted hangings in hospitals do not use a strong enough noose or sufficient drop height to cause death through spinal cord injury. Cerebral hypoxia through asphyxiation is the probable cause of death. Emergency airway management is a priority.

Injury to the soft tissues of the neck (B) may cause respiratory obstruction. Close attention to the development of pulmonary complications is required.

Impaired consciousness (D) is associated with degree of hypoxia but is not directly causative for foot drop.

Aggressive resuscitation and treatment of post-anoxic brain injury (E) is indicated even in patients without evident neurological signs.

25. B ★★★★ OHPsych 3rd edn → pp.964–5

This question asks about the symptoms associated with antidepressant discontinuation syndrome (often called SSRI withdrawal syndrome). Paroxetine (B) is the SSRI with the shortest half-life and hence is associated with the highest risk of withdrawal symptoms from stopping use.

Lithium (A) withdrawal may bring common problems such as feeling anxious, irritable, tense, restless, highly emotional, or confused. There don't seem to be any physical 'rebound phenomena'.

Stopping propranolol (C) can cause irregular heartbeat and a rebound anxiety on withdrawal.

Withdrawal psychosis and tardive dyskinesia are two of the most serious problems caused by withdrawal from antipsychotics such as quetiapine (D).

Temazepam (E) is an intermediate-acting benzodiazepine. Benzodiazepine withdrawal symptoms include anxiety, confusion, hallucinations, insomnia, cold sweats, heart palpitations, tremor, tinnitus, and detachment.

→ NICE Clinical Guideline 90—Depression in adults: http://guidance.nice.org.uk/CG90.

Extended Matching Questions

1. J ★★

The cause of any acute confusional state is multifactorial, so consider the biopsychosocial model. A full history and examination will highlight the likely cause dependent on the clinical scenario. In this case, the age, duration of symptoms, and indication of urinary symptoms make a UTI highly likely.

2. C ★★

Clozapine is an atypical antipsychotic which is known to be effective in treating treatment-resistant schizophrenia but which has a number of life-threatening side-effects, including arrhythmias, myocarditis, cardiomyopathy, pericarditis, and thromboembolism. In this scenario he may well have myocarditis, which usually develops within the first month often as a non-specific fever and with symptoms of an infection before developing into full myocarditis at around five days. Monitoring guidelines advise checking CRP and troponin at baseline and weekly for the first four weeks after clozapine initiation and observing the patient for signs and symptoms of illness.

3. H ★★

Given the presentation of suicidal thoughts and a lack of physical illness, an MSE would be appropriate to look for signs of mental disorder. She is clearly upset and not caring for herself. The presence of a young baby would necessitate a social service referral.

4. D ★★

Ictal, interictal, and post-ictal psychoses are uncommon but important to recognize complications of epilepsy. Bizarre aggressive behaviour can occur without psychosis during a seizure. In this instance, it is possible that this man is attempting to avoid conviction by claiming a medical condition rather than taking responsibility for his aggressive outbursts. Working closely with the police is advisable for all concerned.

5. I ★★

The above constellation of symptoms fit with a picture of hyperthyroidism. There can sometimes be a physical cause for some 'psychiatric' symptoms which when treated can resolve the issues. This patient will need careful follow-up to make sure that her symptoms are related to her thyroid and not also psychological.

General feedback on 1–5: OHPsych 3rd edn → pp.52–8, 150–2

6. F ★★

Post-natal depression occurs in 10–15% of women within six months after birth. The clinical features are similar to usual depression, although thought content may include worries about the baby's health or being an inadequate mother.

7. G ★★

Post-partum PTSD is seen after an excessively tough labour: in particular, where there was intense and prolonged pain, a subjective loss of control or complications requiring emergency caesarean section, or fear of stillbirth. The mother may experience classical PTSD which can last for months. Some women will avoid any further childbirth, or those who are pregnant again may experience further symptoms, especially in the last trimester. Psychological therapy has been shown to help alleviate these symptoms and help prevent their reoccurrence later.

8. I ★★

Puerperal (or post-natal) psychosis is an acute psychotic episode, occurring after 1.5/1000 births, with a peak occurrence at two weeks after birth. Common features include lability of symptoms, insomnia, perplexity, and thoughts of suicide or infanticide. Without treatment they can last for months and may result in serious risk to the baby and mother. Treatment is similar to any psychotic disorder, usually with good results. In some cases, admission is necessary often to a special mother and baby unit. Here, follow-up is important for the current birth and any future pregnancies.

9. A ★★

Up to three-quarters of new mothers experience a short-lived period of tearfulness and emotional lability starting around two days after birth and lasting a few days; this is termed 'baby blues'. These usually resolve and do not develop into full depression or require treatment. If they persist then a referral may be necessary. Recently, there has been mention of 'baby pinks', where new mothers are overly and illogically on top of the world, which is considered a possible precursor to a manic episode.

10. B ★★

BPAD requires at least two episodes of mental illness for diagnosis, one of which must be hypomanic, manic, or mixed. Recovery is usually complete between episodes. In the post-natal period the symptoms of BPAD will be the same as at any other time; however, the treatment may need to take into account breastfeeding and the physiological demands of early motherhood, for example lack of sleep.

General feedback on 6–10: OHPsych 3rd edn → pp.240, 418, 420–1

→ PANDAS (Pre and Postnatal Depression Advice and Support)— http://www.pandasfoundation.org.uk/help-and-information/

pre-ante-and-postnatal-illnesses/baby-blues.html?gclid=CPKf37SwrbkC Fc2_3godi0UApQ#.UiTdjTbD9nQ.

11. A ★★★

Anosognosia is a failure to identify functional deficits caused by an organic disease which usually presents as injury due to inattention. For anosognosia to exist there needs to be a combination of hemiplegia and additional brain injury to produce another deficit. Most often this is found in patients with a stroke. Often it is associated with damage to the temporoparietal junction, although this is not the site that caused the hemiplegia.

12. J ★★★

Simultagnosia is the failure to recognize more than a single object at a time. For the patient, stationary objects disappear from view and then reappear when attention is shifted to them. It can also be demonstrated as a failure to understand the overall meaning of a picture despite being able to understand individual details of the picture. To establish the presence of simultagnosia, the 'Boston Cookie Theft' picture is used. It is associated with bilateral injury at the junction between the occipital and parietal lobes usually from a stroke or traumatic brain injury.

13. B ★★★

Aphasia is a broad term which encompasses many different disturbances of the comprehension and formulation of language. The difficulty here is found in expressive aphasia, where the patient knows what he or she wants to communicate but cannot do so, which slows spoken and written communication, and even sign language. It is associated with damage to Broca's area, hence it being known as Broca's aphasia, and is caused by stroke or traumatic brain injury, most likely an extradural haematoma or cerebral haemorrhage. This form of aphasia should be differentiated from dysarthria, which is an inability to produce understandable speech due to difficulties in movement of the muscles of the mouth and tongue.

14. I ★★★

Prosopagnosia refers to a failure to recognize faces. These can be familiar faces, such as relations or friends, or famous faces, such as the Queen. It is associated with bilateral lesions of the occipitotemporal regions of the brain. In advanced Alzheimer's disease, a patient may develop severe prosopagnosia and fail to recognize themselves in a mirror. It is found following traumatic brain injury and also as a congenital disorder which may affect up to 2.5% of the population.

15. D ★★★

Asterognosia is the failure to identify a three-dimensional object by touch alone. This is something of an interesting finding rather than a patient complaint as it is not often of great importance to the patient. It is associated with lesions of the parietal lobe or dorsal column.

General feedback on 11–15: OHPsych 3rd edn → pp.68–9

→ Sacks O (2010). A neurologist's notebook: face-blind. *The New Yorker*. http://www.newyorker.com/reporting/2010/08/30/100830fa_fact_sacks.

Psychopharmacology

Kazuya Iwata

Psychotropic drugs are the main form of physical treatment in psychiatry and they exert their action by mainly acting on dopamine, noradrenaline, serotonin, and muscarinic receptors.

Antipsychotics, which are the mainline treatment for psychotic illnesses, usually act by blocking dopamine receptors in the dopamine pathways of the brain, usually the mesolimbic system. The D2 receptors are the usual target of the antipsychotics, although clozapine, which is considered the gold standard antipsychotic, has a strong affinity for the D4 receptors. The underlying principle of antipsychotic treatment builds on the dopamine theory of schizophrenia, whereby an excess of dopamine is linked to the development of psychotic symptoms. Overactive dopamine receptors are thought to be involved in this, and thus blockage of the dopamine receptors through antipsychotics can provide relief from psychotic symptoms.

Antipsychotics are divided into typical and atypical, and the defining feature of typicals is their propensity to cause EPSEs. This is thought to be due to the fact that typical antipsychotics are not specific for dopamine receptors in the mesolimbic pathways, but can also block those in mesocortical, tuberoinfundibular, and nigrostriatal pathways.

Atypical antipsychotics can impact on a variety of receptor types, such as serotonin, and thus they are usually subclassified according to their pharmacological properties. Their heterogeneous pharmacodynamics in part explains their variable side-effect profile. One common side-effect of atypical antipsychotics is their tendency to trigger metabolic syndrome, which is a cluster of cardiovascular risk factors including dyslipidaemia, hypertension, central obesity, and impaired glucose tolerance. They also cause endocrine-related side-effects, such as hyperprolactinaemia.

An important adverse effect seen with any antipsychotic is neuroleptic malignant syndrome (NMS), which is an idiosyncratic reaction to antipsychotics taken even at therapeutic doses. Patients can present with hyperthermia, rigidity, autonomic disturbances, and altered mental state over 24–48 hours. It can be potentially life threatening, and thus, if suspected, urgent referral to a general hospital is required.

Antidepressants also vary greatly with regards to their pharmacological properties, but the majority increase the concentration of neurotransmitters in the synaptic cleft to alleviate depressive symptoms. The main classes are serotonin reuptake inhibitors, tricyclic antidepressants, serotonin and noradrenaline reuptake inhibitors, MAOIs, and noradrenaline and specific serotonergic antidepressants. The side-effect profile therefore depends on the receptors affected: antimuscarinic effects include blurred vision and urinary retention; antihistaminergic effects include drowsiness; and anti-adrenergic effects include postural hypotension and arrhythmia. There can also be life-threatening side-effects with the use of some antidepressants, and these include hypertensive crisis when tyramine-containing food is ingested whilst on MAOIs, and serotonin syndrome if the concentration of serotonin reaches a dangerous level through overdose on serotonergic medications.

When commencing patients on any psychotropic medication, it is important that they are monitored regularly, including carrying out relevant investigations. Some medications like lithium and clozapine require regular blood tests, and it is always good to screen for any metabolic side-effects.

Kazuya Iwata

QUESTIONS

Single Best Answers

1. A 27-year-old woman with schizophrenia is informed that she will be treated with quetiapine. She is told this is an atypical antipsychotic and better than typicals, but does not understand what this means. Which is the *single* most appropriate explanation to give her regarding these types of antipsychotics? ★

A Antipsychotics available as oral and depot solutions are designated as typical, while atypicals exist as oral solution

B Antipsychotics developed before 1960 are classified as typical, while those developed after 1961 are atypical

C Atypical antipsychotics are characterized by the presence of an aliphatic chain in their molecular structure

D Atypical antipsychotics have a lower propensity to cause EPSEs compared to typical antipsychotics

E Typical antipsychotics are primarily effective for psychotic disorders, while atypical antipsychotics are effective for both psychotic and affective illnesses

2. A 29-year-old man with schizophrenia is commenced on olanzapine. Two hours later he becomes stiff in his neck and says that his jaw is rigid. Which is the *single* most appropriate initial management? ★

A Change his antipsychotic to a typical agent like haloperidol

B Emergency treatment with procyclidine

C Give a test dose of zuclopenthixol injection

D Offer analgesia such as ibuprofen or paracetamol

E Transfer to hospital for suspected NMS

3. A 36-year-old woman with BPAD is taking lithium. She developed lithium toxicity after starting a medication that her GP prescribed for a medical problem. Which is the *single* most likely medication to have contributed to this? ★

A Erythromycin

B Indometacin

C Lansoprazole

D Paracetamol

E Theophylline

4. A 29-year-old man with treatment-resistant schizophrenia is being considered for a trial of clozapine therapy. He is 'needle-phobic' and would like to know what regular investigations are needed while taking clozapine. Which is the *single* most appropriate answer to give? ★

A Full blood count

B Glucose

C Kidney function test

D Liver function test

E Thyroid function test

5. A 30-year-old man with schizophrenia is commenced on olanzapine. Which is the *single* most appropriate set of side-effects that this man should be warned about? ★

A Dyslipidaemia and obesity

B Hypercortisolaemia and 'moon facing'

C Hyperprolactinaemia and increased insulin secretion

D Hypochromic anaemia and dizziness

E Hypothyroidism and deranged kidney function

6. A 46-year-old woman with BPAD develops lithium toxicity despite taking her regular dose of medication. Which is the *single* most appropriate contributory factor to her toxicity? ★

A Gout

B Heavy smoking

C Hyperthyroidism

D Kidney failure

E Liver failure

7. A 16-year-old adolescent has had a low mood, low energy drive, and constant thoughts of ending her life for eight months despite attending regular psychotherapy and receiving community support. Which is the *single* most appropriate medication to prescribe? ★★

A Citalopram

B Fluoxetine

C Lithium

D Valproate

E Venlafaxine

8. A 35-year-old man with schizoaffective disorder develops hyperkinesia, hyperreflexia, and hyperthermia within hours of starting a new treatment regimen. His muscles are moderately rigid. Which is the *single* most likely diagnosis? ★★

A Antidepressant-induced hyponatraemia

B 'Cheese reaction'

C EPSE

D Neuroleptic malignant syndrome

E Serotonin syndrome

9. A 10-year-old boy with attention deficit hyperactivity disorder is commenced on a first-line medication and shows subsequent improvement in his behaviours. Which is the *single* most appropriate pharmacological explanation that would explain his improvement? ★★

A Antagonistic effect on D2 and D4 receptors result in suppression of hyperactivity

B Enhancement of GABA transmission to reduce neuronal firing and induce a calming effect

C Increased release of dopamine and noradrenaline triggers a paradoxical increase in concentration

D Inhibition of serotonin and noradrenaline reuptake leads to decreased impulsivity

E Modification of N-methyl-D-aspartate (NMDA) and GABA receptors exert an inhibitory effect to improve attention

10. A 35-year-old man with schizophrenia is commenced on clozapine by his psychiatrist. He has read on the internet that this drug is most effective when combined with lifestyle changes. Which is the *single* most appropriate advice to give him? ★★

A Avoid cheese and pickled herring

B Commence regular exercise

C Cut down on smoking

D Refrain from having unprotected sexual intercourse

E Sleep at least six hours at set times

11. A 20-year-old man develops priapism two weeks after starting a medication for depression. Which is the *single* medication most likely to be responsible for this? ★★★

A Fluoxetine

B Mirtazapine

C St John's wort

D Trazodone

E Venlafaxine

12. A 48-year-old woman with schizophrenia who was previously alert becomes mute and immobile. She is taking risperidone. Which is the *single* most appropriate initial treatment? ★★★

A Increase her risperidone dose

B Prescribe high-dose fluoxetine

C Prescribe lorazepam

D Prescribe procyclidine

E Switch risperidone to clozapine

13. A 32-year-old woman with BPAD has been treated with lithium. She has continued to take lithium until discovering she was 24 weeks pregnant. She is concerned that there may have been side-effects for the fetus. Which is the *single* most relevant side-effect to discuss with her? ★★★

A Coarctation of the aorta with heart failure

B Downward displacement of the tricuspid valve

C Left to right shunt with pulmonary hypertension

D Patent ductus and failure to thrive

E Right ventricular hypertrophy and interventricular defect

14. A 29-year-old man is having relationship problems with his wife since commencing fluoxetine eight weeks ago. Which is the *single* most likely mechanism by which fluoxetine may be responsible? ★★★

A Decreased inhibition

B Erectile dysfunction

C Gynaecomastia

D Hypersexuality

E Increased irritability

15. A 37-year-old man with atypical depression is commenced on moclobemide and develops headaches, papilloedema, and severe anxiety. He has not had cheese, yeast extracts, or alcohol but has used nasal decongestants for his hay fever. Which is the *single* most appropriate explanation for his symptoms? ★★★

A Antihistaminergic effect of the decongestant triggering monoamine crisis

B Development of cerebral oedema following moclobemide overdose

C Hypertensive crisis triggered by sympathomimetics in decongestants

D Idiopathic allergic reaction to moclobemide resulting in malignant hyperthermia

E Raised cortisol from decongestant leading to adrenal crisis

16. A 36-year-old woman with a relapse of schizoaffective disorder has recently given birth to a baby boy and wishes to breastfeed him. Which is the *single* most appropriate medication to prescribe her safely? ★★★

A Chlorpromazine

B Clozapine

C Lithium

D Moclobemide

E Risperidone

17. A 28-year-old man with schizophrenia is commenced on clozapine, having been unresponsive to olanzapine, haloperidol, and aripiprazole. Which is the *single* most appropriate description of the primary mode of action of this new medication? ★★★★

A Antagonistic effects on 5HT2 receptor, with some D2 affinity

B Antagonistic effects on all dopamine receptors (D1–5)

C Antagonistic effects on D1 and D4 receptors

D Antagonistic effects on D2 receptor

E Mechanism unknown

18. A 28-year-old woman has had epilepsy for a number of years. This has been previously well treated with sodium valproate and she has shown good compliance. Recently she was admitted to hospital following a deterioration in her mental state and she is additionally diagnosed with schizophrenia. Which is the *single* most appropriate treatment? ★★★★

A Clozapine alone to treat both epilepsy and schizophrenia

B Haloperidol should be considered depending on tolerability

C High-dose chlorpromazine as a trial regime

D Increase dose of her anticonvulsant to trigger mood-stabilizing effects

E Olanzapine as first-line antipsychotic treatment

19. A 22-year-old woman with depression is commenced on fluoxetine, and her psychiatrist advises her that the medication can take up to eight weeks to be fully effective. Which is the *single* most appropriate mechanism that accounts for this delayed onset of action? ★★★★

A Downregulation of post-synaptic receptors and desensitization of pre-synaptic autoreceptors

B Inhibition of both serotonin and noradrenaline reuptake pumps

C Poor absorption of fluoxetine metabolites from the gut

D Slow rewiring of the neuronal circuitry in the limbic system

E Upregulation of post-synaptic serotonin receptors coupled to G-proteins

20. A 65-year-old man with chronic Parkinson's disease becomes psychotic and requires treatment. However, his wife is concerned about antipsychotics possibly exacerbating his parkinsonism. Which is the *single* most appropriate treatment? ★★★★

A Clozapine

B ECT

C Haloperidol

D Increase levodopa dose

E Zuclopenthixol injection

Extended Matching Questions

Investigations

For each scenario below, choose the *single* most appropriate investigation indicated in the given scenario from the list of options. Each option may be used once, more than once, or not at all. ★

A   Blood pressure

B   Blood sugar

C   Creatinine kinase

D   Dopamine level

E   Lipid profile

F   Liver function tests

G   Platelet count

H   Prolactin level

I   Serum level of medication

J   Thyroid function test

1. A 20-year-old man with schizophrenia is commenced on clozapine at a therapeutic dose. As he remains unsettled, his psychiatrist orders an investigation.

2. A 27-year-old woman with BPAD is having her medication changed from lithium to carbamazepine. Her psychiatrist orders an investigation prior to changing the medication.

3. A 28-year-old woman with schizoaffective disorder has been treated with venlafaxine, and she is now being given the maximum dose. Her psychiatrist asks her GP to monitor her regularly.

4. A 30-year-old man newly diagnosed with schizophrenia is given haloperidol and develops fever and muscular rigidity. NMS is suspected, and an investigation is ordered to confirm the diagnosis.

5. A 36-year-old woman is newly diagnosed with BPAD. She requires an investigation prior to starting lithium and a repeat every six to twelve months.

Side-effects

For each scenario below, choose the *single* most appropriate side-effect likely to be seen in the given scenario from the list of options. Each option may be used once, more than once, or not at all. ★

A Acute dystonia

B Agranulocytosis

C Hypercortisolaemia

D Hyperprolactinaemia

E Liver failure

F Malignant hyperthermia

G Nephropathy

H Serotonin syndrome

I Stevens–Johnson's syndrome

J Tardive dyskinesia

6. A 28-year-old man with schizoaffective disorder has been taking risperidone for two months. He is mentally stable but feels that the medication is affecting his 'personal life' too much.

7. A 30-year-old woman newly diagnosed with BPAD is commenced on carbamazepine but is taken to hospital within hours of taking it because of an acute reaction. Her FBC is normal.

8. A 31-year-old woman newly diagnosed with schizophrenia is given haloperidol. An hour later, she develops a side-effect which is relieved when given an anticholinergic agent.

9. A 45-year-old woman with BPAD has been settled on lithium for over ten years. Her psychiatrist has decided to change her mood stabilizer due to this side-effect.

10. A 55-year-old man with schizophrenia has been on a stable dose of chlorpromazine for over 20 years, but his psychiatrist has discontinued it because he felt that he was developing an irreversible side-effect.

ANSWERS

Single Best Answers

1. D ★   OHPsych 3rd edn → pp.200–4

The greatest distinguishing factor between the two classes of antipsychotics is the propensity to trigger EPSEs (D), which encompasses movement disorders such as akathisia, dystonia, parkinsonism, and tardive dyskinesia. When explaining this to the patient it is important to use clear, jargon-free language and pitch the explanation to the appropriate level for her understanding.

Both typical and atypical antipsychotics exist in oral and depot solutions (A).

Although the majority of the typicals are older and atypicals are newer, this is not always the case; for example, clozapine is an atypical antipsychotic which was developed in the 1950s (B).

Aliphatic compounds are compounds of carbon and hydrogen which do not contain benzene or similarly aromatic rings. The presence of aliphatic chains has no bearing on the distinction between typical and atypical antipsychotics (C).

Both antipsychotic types are effective against psychotic symptoms, and can be used in treating affective illnesses such as BPAD and schizoaffective disorder. However, this is not a factor that distinguishes the two types of antipsychotics (E).

2. B ★   OHPsych 3rd edn → pp.954–5

The patient described here displays signs suggestive of acute dystonia, which is one of the EPSEs. Anticholinergic agents such as procyclidine are effective in relieving these symptoms (B).

Changing an atypical antipsychotic to a typical agent like haloperidol (A) can increase the likelihood of developing further EPSEs.

There is no indication of introducing a depot antipsychotic in the given situation (C).

If the patient is in discomfort, analgesics may be offered (D), but the most appropriate treatment is the use of anticholinergics to treat the underlying cause of the stiffness.

Development of severe rigidity following the use of antipsychotics is an indication of possible NMS (E), but the given clinical description matches that of acute dystonia. Patients with suspected NMS would tend to develop symptoms over 24–48 hours and will be unwell with hyperthermia, diaphoresis, and altered consciousness.

3. B ★   OHPsych 3rd edn → pp.336–40

The most likely medication is indometacin (B). NSAIDs such as indometacin can reduce the excretion of lithium by the kidneys, and thus concomitant use can lead to increased serum levels of lithium. Care should be taken when analgesics are prescribed, and patients should be encouraged to take plenty of fluids.

Erythromycin is a hepatic enzyme inhibitor, but as lithium is not metabolized by the liver, it would have no bearing on serum lithium levels (A).

Antacids such as lansoprazole (C) increase excretion of lithium and thus would lead to lower serum levels.

Paracetamol (D) does not have any effect on lithium levels.

Theophylline (E) increases excretion of lithium and thus would lower serum levels.

4. A ★   OHPsych 3rd edn → pp.212–13

One of the potential side-effects of clozapine use is agranulocytosis, resulting in leucopaenia and possible death. In order to avoid this, clozapine can only be prescribed if the patient's FBC (A), especially neutrophils, is regularly monitored. Blood tests are initially done weekly but can be gradually spaced out to monthly testing.

Although glucose intolerance is a potential outcome of long-term use of atypical antipsychotics such as clozapine, it is not the most important blood test that is required on a regular basis (B).

It is always good to monitor the patient's general physical health, but kidney function testing is not required regularly for clozapine therapy (C).

LFTs (D) should be done at least every six to twelve months in conjunction with a lipid profile, but it is not required regularly for clozapine therapy. It is indicated when treating patients with mood stabilizers.

Regular monitoring of thyroid function is required for patients on lithium therapy (E).

5. A ★   OHPsych 3rd edn → pp.934–5

The answer is dyslipidaemia and obesity (A). Atypical antipsychotics, such as olanzapine, have a propensity to trigger metabolic syndrome, which consists of hypertension, dyslipidaemia (including hypercholesterolaemia), central obesity, and raised plasma fasting glucose.

Hypercortisolaemia and 'moon facing' (B) would suggest a diagnosis of Cushing's disease. This is not a recognized complication of olanzapine

Olanzapine can occasionally lead to hyperprolactinaemia (C) but only rarely causes clinical manifestations. This is often seen in risperidone instead. In addition, the use of atypicals tends to trigger glucose dysregulation.

Hypochromic anaemia (D) is not a common manifestation of olanzapine, although it can rarely cause leucopaenia.

Hypothyroidism and deranged kidney function (E) are usually seen with long-term usage of lithium, not olanzapine.

6. D ★   OHPsych 3rd edn → pp.338–9

As the majority of lithium is excreted by the kidneys, kidney failure (D) can lead to decreased lithium excretion and may contribute to the development of lithium toxicity. Lithium toxicity can present with marked tremors, anorexia, nausea, and lethargy in early stages; in severe cases it can cause restlessness, muscle fasciculation, ataxia, dysarthria, delirium, and coma.

Gout (A) is not usually linked to lithium toxicity.

Heavy smoking (B) can alter the concentration of serum clozapine, but will not affect lithium levels.

Lithium is known to cause goitre (an enlarged thyroid) and can lead to the development of thyroid dysfunction such as hyperthyroidism or hypothyroidism, but its excretion is not affected by the patient's thyroid status. In fact, lithium can be used in those with thyroid disorders as long as their thyroid disorder is treated and reviewed regularly.

Only a negligible amount of lithium is excreted by the digestive system, and thus the impact of liver failure (E) would not be significant on the development of lithium toxicity.

7. B ★★   OHPsych 3rd edn → pp.652–3

Fluoxetine (B) is the recommended first-line antidepressant for adolescents according to NICE guidelines, as it has a favourable risk:benefit ratio.

Citalopram (A) is used in treating adolescent depression, but usually as a second-line treatment.

Lithium (C) can be used to treat BPAD in adolescents, but there is no indication that this patient suffers from a manic presentation.

Valproate (D) can be used to treat BPAD in adolescents, but is usually not given to women due to its teratogenic effects. Also there is no indication in this scenario that the patient has BPAD.

Venlafaxine (E) is generally avoided in adolescents, as the risks of hostility, suicidal ideations, and self-harm are thought to outweigh its clinical benefits.

8. E ★★   OHPsych 3rd edn → pp.960–2

The answer is serotonin syndrome (E). This can present with autonomic dysfunction, rigidity, hyperthermia, and altered mental state which can be rapid in onset and progression. Its presentation is similar to NMS but is marked by less severe muscle rigidity, hyperkinesias, and having serotonergic agents as its aetiology. In this scenario the patient probably had an unintentional overdose.

Antidepressants, in particular SSRIs, can trigger hyponatraemia (A) and this is thought to be due to the syndrome of inappropriate secretion of antidiuretic hormone (ADH). The presentation will depend on the degree of hyponatraemia, and can include findings such as lethargy, confusion, muscle weakness, and hypertension.

The 'cheese reaction' (B) is seen with the ingestion of tyramine-containing food material while taking MAOIs. This results in a hypertensive crisis, manifesting with headaches, papilloedema, dyspnoea, and arrhythmia.

EPSEs (C) are seen with antipsychotics, usually typical, and include motor problems such as tardive dyskinesia, dystonia, and akathisia. EPSEs do not include symptoms such as hyperthermia and hyperreflexia.

NMS (D) is an idiosyncratic reaction to antipsychotics and is characterized by fever, severe muscle rigidity, bradykinesia, hyperthermia, and autonomic dysfunction. It can take several days to develop.

9. C ★★ OHPsych 3rd edn → pp.628–9

Methylphenidate is the preferred treatment for ADHD. Like amphetamines, it acts on the dopamine transporter and noradrenaline transporter proteins to inhibit their reuptake. The increased dopamine levels, and to a lesser extent increased noradrenaline, are thought to increase concentration and attention in treated children (C).

Antagonistic activities of D2 and D4 receptors are seen in antipsychotics. They are not involved in methylphenidate's actions to suppress hyperactivity (A).

Enhancing GABA transmission to decrease neuronal excitability is the underlying mechanism for benzodiazepines, not methylphenidate (B).

Inhibition of serotonin and noradrenaline reuptake are seen in antidepressants such as venlafaxine. They are not involved in methylphenidate's actions to decrease impulsivity (D).

Methylphenidate is not recognized to have an effect on NMDA or GABA receptors (E).

10. C ★★ OHPsych 3rd edn → pp.210–11

Cigarette smoking can significantly increase the clearance of clozapine, thus reducing plasma concentration and subsequently its efficacy. Patients who smoke should be encouraged to decrease, or better stop, their smoking (C).

Advice to avoid cheese and pickled herring (A) should be given to patients commencing MAOIs in order to prevent the 'cheese' reaction, which is a dangerous rise in BP following ingestion of tyramine-containing food.

Clozapine may trigger metabolic syndrome, and so regular exercise (B) and healthy eating should be encouraged, but this will not directly affect the effectiveness of clozapine.

Unprotected intercourse (D) should be discouraged in patients who are at risk of sexually transmitted infections, but this has no effect on clozapine efficacy.

Good sleep hygiene (E) is useful to ensure that the patient does not miss their medication times, but it will not directly affect clozapine efficacy. Patients with schizophrenia, depression, anxiety, and BPAD may all experience difficulty sleeping, so sleep hygiene advice can be an important aspect of managing mental illnesses.

11. D ★★★ OHPsych 3rd edn → pp.942–3

Priapism is a rare but potentially serious side-effect of trazodone (D). Approximately 80% of all cases of drug-induced priapism are thought to be due to trazodone, and if this is suspected the medication needs to be stopped immediately. Blockade of α1-adrenergic receptors is thought to be responsible for this.

Fluoxetine (A) may cause sexual side-effects, such as erectile dysfunction and decreased libido, but not priapism.

Sexual side-effects are not usually seen with mirtazapine (B).

St John's wort (C) is an unlicensed, 'herbal remedy' for mild depression. It has serotonergic effects and may interact with other medications.

Venlafaxine (E) may cause sexual side-effects such as decreased libido, impotence, or difficulty having an orgasm. However, priapism is not usually associated with venlafaxine use.

12. C ★★★ OHPsych 3rd edn → pp.992–3

Benzodiazepines such as lorazepam (C) are an effective treatment for catatonic presentations and have a good evidence base in successfully treating 70–80% of cases. An alternative would be the use of ECT.

Reviewing the patient's antipsychotic medication is something that should be done when the presentation changes, but increasing the medication is not necessarily indicated here in the first instance (A). Catatonia-like presentation can also be seen in NMS and thus changes in antipsychotic doses need to be made with caution.

Fluoxetine is an SSRI used in treating depressive symptoms. The patient in this scenario is suffering from catatonia as opposed to depression, and thus fluoxetine is not indicated here (B).

Anticholinergic agents such as procyclidine (D) are used in treating EPSEs which can cause feelings of 'stiffness', but anticholinergic agents are not indicated in treating catatonia.

The need for clozapine is not indicated here as an initial treatment (E).

13. B ★★★ OHPsych 3rd edn → pp.338–9

Downward displacement of the tricuspid valve (B) is the most relevant side-effect. This is Ebstein's anomaly, and the risk is increased with maternal use of lithium during the first trimester. The risk is said to be increased eight-fold.

Coarctation of the aorta with heart failure (A) is a type of congenital atrial septal defect, but not usually linked to lithium.

Left to right shunt with pulmonary hypertension (C) is Eisenmenger's syndrome, a congenital heart defect, but not usually linked to lithium.

Patent ductus and failure to thrive (D) is a type of congenital atrial septal defect, but not usually linked to lithium.

Right ventricular hypertrophy and interventricular defect (E) is not the correct answer. The symptoms described here are part of Fallot's tetralogy, which also include overriding aorta and pulmonary stenosis. It is not usually linked to lithium.

14. B ★★★   OHPsych 3rd edn → pp.478–9

Sexual side-effects, including erectile dysfunction (B), decreased libido, and anorgasmia, are commonly seen with the use of SSRIs.

Decreased inhibition (A) is not a recognized side-effect of fluoxetine.

Gynaecomastia (C) can be due to hyperprolactinaemia, which can be triggered by risperidone, and may cause discomfort in men. However, it is not associated with fluoxetine.

Hypersexuality (D) is not a recognized side-effect of fluoxetine, although hypersexuality and pathological gambling are seen with the use of dopamine receptor agonists (e.g. pramipexole) used in the treatment of parkinsonism.

Increased irritability (E) is not a recognized side-effect of fluoxetine.

15. C ★★★   OHPsych 3rd edn → pp.272–3

Sympathomimetics in nasal decongestants can trigger a hypertensive crisis (C), just like any foodstuff containing tyramine, such as cheese and pickled herring, when on an MAOI. This is a potential fatal side-effect and thus patients need to be warned about potential substances that can trigger this interaction.

There is no evidence linking nasal decongestants with monoamine crisis (A).

Overdose in moclobemide is considered to be less toxic and is generally preferred in those who are at risk of taking an overdose (B).

Malignant hyperthermia is a potentially life-threatening condition that can develop as a result of exposure to general anaesthesia, and can present with hyperthermia, tachypnoea, and tachycardia. It is not related to moclobemide (D).

There is no evidence linking nasal decongestants to development of adrenal crisis (E).

16. A ★★★   OHPsych 3rd edn → pp.970–1

Prescribing in lactation should always be done cautiously, as there will always be a risk of the active substance being transferred to the infant. The level of antipsychotics in the infant is said to be low to undetectable, but caution should still be exercised. Typical antipsychotics, such as chlorpromazine (A) and haloperidol, are recommended for use with caution.

Clozapine (B) should be actively avoided in breastfeeding due to the potential effects of agranulocytosis in the infant.

Lithium (C) should be actively avoided in breastfeeding due to its potential effects on the infant's kidneys and thyroid.

MAOIs like moclobemide are not recommended for use in breastfeeding (D).

Although levels of antipsychotics in breast milk may be low, *typical* antipsychotics are recommended, rather than *atypical* antipsychotics such as risperidone (E). This is due to the amount of evidence available at this time.

17. C ★★★★   OHPsych 3rd edn → pp.210–11

The answer is (C). Clozapine acts as an antagonist on D1 and D4 receptors, and has very little affinity for D2.

The involvement of 5HT2 and D2 receptors (A) is seen in atypical antipsychotics such as olanzapine, risperidone, and quetiapine.

Antagonistic effects on all dopamine receptors (D1–5) is the mode of action for haloperidol (B).

Most antipsychotics have some antagonistic effect on D2 receptor (D), apart from clozapine which has less affinity to it.

The mechanism of action of clozapine is understood (antagonistic effect on D1 and D4 receptors). However, the exact mechanism by which lithium works is still unknown (E).

18. B ★★★★   OHPsych 3rd edn → pp.978–9

Haloperidol should be considered depending on tolerability (B). Both haloperidol and quetiapine are associated with the lowest risk with regards to lowering seizure threshold, and thus it is reasonable to consider either of these as an antipsychotic for those with pre-existing epilepsy. A seizure threshold is the balance of excitatory and inhibitory forces in the brain which affects one's susceptibility to seizures. Patients taking medications that lower this threshold are more susceptible to seizures.

Clozapine alone to treat both epilepsy and schizophrenia (A) is not the most appropriate treatment. Antipsychotics such as olanzapine, chlorpromazine, and clozapine can lower the seizure threshold and thus should be avoided in patients with epilepsy.

High-dose chlorpromazine as a trial regime (C) is not the most appropriate treatment. Anti-epileptic medications such as sodium valproate are used as mood stabilizers, but are not indicated as first-line treatment of schizophrenia. This patient needs a separate antipsychotic medication in the first instance.

Increasing the dose of her anticonvulsant to trigger mood-stabilizing effects (D) would also not be appropriate. Also, reducing this patient's sodium valproate dose would worsen her epilepsy control and would have no beneficial effect on treating her psychotic symptoms.

Clozapine is not routinely offered as a first-line treatment of schizophrenia (E), and its propensity to lower the seizure threshold would not make it a suitable treatment.

19. A ★★★★ OHPsych 3rd edn → pp.266–7

Downregulation of post-synaptic receptors and desensitization of pre-synaptic autoreceptors (A) is the most appropriate mechanism. The initial blockade of serotonin reuptake pumps by fluoxetine leads to an increase in the concentration of serotonin in the synaptic cleft. This triggers a chain of adaptive responses in the neurons, including desensitization of pre-synaptic autoreceptors and post-synaptic serotonin receptors. This is thought to take weeks to complete, and leads to an altered serotonin/receptor ratio, which appears to alleviate depressive symptoms.

Fluoxetine is an SSRI and does not exert its primary effect on noradrenaline receptors (B).

There is no evidence that fluoxetine is poorly absorbed from the gut (C). Peak plasma concentrations are reached six to eight hours after ingestion.

The limbic system is thought to be the part of the brain associated with emotions and memories. There is no evidence that fluoxetine causes rewiring of this neuronal circuitry (D).

The clinical efficacy of SSRIs such as fluoxetine is linked to the downregulation of post-synaptic serotonin receptors, and not upregulation (E).

20. A ★★★★ OHPsych 3rd edn → pp.168–9

In addition to treatment-resistant schizophrenia, clozapine is a recognized treatment for psychotic symptoms seen with Parkinson's disease (A). Its use does not seem to worsen the motor symptoms.

Although ECT can be used in the treatment for neurological crises including extreme Parkinson symptoms, it is not used as first-line treatment (B).

Treatment with antipsychotics such as haloperidol (C) can potentially exacerbate motor symptoms of Parkinson's disease due to its action on the dopamine receptors.

Increasing the dose of levodopa (D) would lead to raised dopamine levels, which in turn may exacerbate his psychotic symptoms.

Not only may the use of depot antipsychotics such as zuclopenthixol (E) exacerbate his parkinsonism, but also it would be difficult to reverse zuclopenthixol's effects as the active substance would remain in the body for longer.

Extended Matching Questions

1. I ★

In patients who are not responding to clozapine despite being prescribed therapeutic doses, serum clozapine levels should be measured. Serum clozapine levels are usually low due to non-compliance or fast metabolism of the drug, for example due to smoking or the presence of liver enzyme inducers.

2. F ★

Carbamazepine and most other anticonvulsants used as mood stabilizers can trigger abnormalities in liver function (including cholangitis and hepatocellular necrosis), and thus LFTs should be carried out prior to starting the medication and around once every three months.

3. A ★

Venlafaxine can trigger hypertension when given at higher doses, and thus patients who are given 200 mg or more should have their BP monitored regularly. There is some evidence that this could be dose-dependent.

4. C ★

NMS is a potentially life-threatening condition, which is thought to be an idiosyncratic reaction to antipsychotics. It is characterized by fever, muscular rigidity, and autonomic dysfunction. Increased CK and urinary myoglobin (due to rhabdomyolysis) support its diagnosis.

5. J ★

Due to its effect on the thyroid and kidneys, urea and electrolytes (U&Es) and TFTs should be checked prior to commencing the medication. Thereafter U&Es and lithium levels are checked every three months, and TFTs should be repeated every six to twelve months.

General feedback on 1–5: OHPsych 3rd edn → pp.278–9, 336–7, 956–66

6. D ★

Certain antipsychotics, notably risperidone, have the propensity to raise prolactin levels. This can manifest as loss of sexual interest and impotence in men, and amenorrhoea and galactorrhoea in women. Care should be given when prescribing to younger adults.

7. I ★

Carbamazepine can trigger Stevens–Johnson's syndrome in some patients, and as blood results can usually be normal, they need to be monitored for signs of its early development. Stevens–Johnson's syndrome is a form of toxic epidermal necrolysis and manifests as ulcers and skin lesions, initially in mucous membranes but gradually spreading to the rest of the body. It can develop rapidly, from within hours after first contact with the trigger.

8. A ★

Typical antipsychotics can manifest with EPSEs, which is a collection of side-effects consisting of parkinsonism, akathisia, acute dystonia, and tardive dyskinesia. Acute dystonia is the development of muscle spasms, commonly involving the neck, jaws, and back, and can develop acutely following contact with typical antipsychotics. They are usually relieved by using anticholinergic agents such as procyclidine and benztropine.

9. G ★

Nephropathy, which includes interstitial fibrosis and tubular atrophy, is seen in patients on long-term lithium therapy, with renal failure being a recognized complication. It is important to monitor kidney function of patients on lithium due to its effect on the kidneys, and also because it is excreted by the kidneys.

10. J ★

Tardive dyskinesia is an EPSE that involves involuntary and repetitive movements of the tongue, lips, and jaw. It occurs after long-term treatment with typical antipsychotics. It can be severe and unresponsive to treatment and may be exacerbated with the use of anticholinergic agents.

General feedback on 6–10: OHPsych 3rd edn → pp.338–47, 942–55

Chapter 7

Psychological treatment and psychotherapy

Esra Caglar

Psychological therapies are often the first-line treatments for psychiatric disorders, depending on their nature and severity. In many cases they work best in conjunction with medication. The UK government is encouraging improved and timely access to psychological treatments in both primary and secondary care services. Psychological treatments can be carried out in community mental health services, specialist psychotherapy services, and the private sector.

Psychological therapies have a rich history. Today a number of evidence-based, innovative treatments are available. There is advanced research in psychotherapy, which comes with its own challenges.

Psychotherapies can be delivered to individuals, families, couples, or groups. They can be as short as a few sessions or can last for more than a year, depending on the modality. The focus may be varied, such as anxiety symptoms, specific phobias, relationship problems, mood disturbances, or difficult life events.

Psychodynamic psychotherapy gives people a fixed time to think—and talk—about the feelings we all have about ourselves and other people such as family or close ones. CBT focuses on how we think about the things going on in our life—thoughts, images, beliefs, and attitudes (cognitive processes)—and how this impacts the way we behave and deal with emotional problems. Family therapy looks at the family as a system and works on each individual's relationship with others and involvement with the problem.

Esra Caglar

QUESTIONS

Single Best Answers

1. A 29-year-old woman has been low in mood for the last two months. She feels tired, has difficulties in concentrating, and feels hopeless about the future. Alongside medication, her GP recommends talking therapy. Which is the *single* most appropriate type of therapy to recommend? ★

A CBT

B Dance movement therapy

C Music therapy

D Play therapy

E Psychodrama

2. A 16-year-old adolescent with excessive weight loss, amenorrhoea, and intense fear of gaining weight comes to the appointment with her parents and elder sister. She says she is just worried about her upcoming GCSE exams. Which is the *single* most appropriate psychological treatment to recommend? ★

A Attachment-based therapy

B CBT

C Dialectic behavioural therapy (DBT)

D Family therapy

E Individual psychodynamic psychotherapy

3. A 35-year-old man had his first panic attack seven months ago whilst presenting a report to a large group at work. Since then, these attacks have increased in frequency and severity and are causing him great distress and limiting his life. He is diagnosed with social anxiety disorder. Group therapy is suggested. Which is the *single* most appropriate description of this type of therapy? ★

A Competition between members is encouraged so that everyone is motivated

B Confidentiality is disregarded so that everyone shares experiences

C Problems with progress are hidden so that nobody is upset

D Silence is discouraged so that everyone interacts verbally

E Spotting mistakes in others is promoted so that everyone learns from them

4. A 19-year-old woman has a history of self-harm and eating disorder. She is seen by a male university counsellor. She says he is the first person she has felt able to open up to and nobody else has understood her as much. She says he is special. He feels good about being revered by his patient. When he discusses this with a colleague, they suggest that this is a countertransference reaction. Which is the *single* most appropriate response to this type of reaction? ★

A Challenge the patient to interpret their feelings immediately

B Enjoy the praise without reflection about the patient's meaning

C Keep these statements confidential from the MDT

D Refuse to see that patient again

E Use these feelings as a tool to understand the patient_

5. A 27-year-old woman is admitted following an overdose. She recently divorced and felt overwhelmed by the situation. She is complimentary about her consultant and his care but has made a complaint about a nurse. At ward round, the charge nurse feels that this woman is wasting their time as an inpatient. The consultant feels sorry for her and thinks a therapist should see her urgently for talking therapy. The charge nurse and consultant have a heated argument over her case. Which *single* psychological defence mechanism is likely to be occurring? ★

A Idealization

B Projective identification

C Rationalization

D Splitting —

E Sublimation

6. A 35-year-old woman has long-term relationship problems, low self-esteem, and a history of childhood trauma. She has been referred to individual psychodynamic psychotherapy and would like to know a little more about what it involves. Which is the *single* most appropriate information to tell her? ★★

A Homework is given at the end of each session

B It is usually limited to eight to twelve sessions

C Reactions and feelings towards the therapist are thought about

D The length of each session will vary

E The patient lies on a couch with the therapist sitting behind —

7. A 47-year-old man spends three hours a day washing his hands. He is very anxious and does not use public toilets, to avoid contamination. He washes all his clothes every time he goes out of the house. The therapist suggests exposure response prevention techniques as part of his therapy. The patient would like to know more before agreeing to this therapy. Which is the *single* main focus for this therapy? ★★

A Childhood experiences that mirror current fears

B Experiments conducted with real objects or stimuli

C Exposure to the fear until it disappears entirely

D Hierarchical list of anxiety-provoking stimuli

E Practising exposure during the sessions only to avoid becoming overwhelmed

8. A 47-year-old man has prostatic cancer with a poor prognosis due to skeletal metastases. At a clinic appointment four months ago, he was told that the ten-year survival rate is 10%. Today in clinic he appears very low in mood and is diagnosed with a severe depressive illness. Which is the *single* most appropriate management? ★★

A CBT

B Gestalt therapy

C Grief counselling

D Psychodynamic psychotherapy

E SSRIs

9. A 26-year-old man receives CBT for his social anxiety. He describes a social gathering of work colleagues where his heart was racing, he felt hot and sweaty, and was light-headed. He said he was very anxious. Afterwards, he wrote down the following thoughts that he remembered having at the time: 'I don't know anyone very well', 'I've got body odour', 'I'm going to faint and make a fool of myself', and 'They will think I am very boring and they will never want to see me again'. Which *single* concept most accurately describes the list of thoughts? ★★

A Core beliefs

B Mentalization

C Negative automatic thoughts

D Reciprocal thoughts

E Underlying assumptions

10. A 16-year-old adolescent has PTSD and repeated DSH. She begins a treatment programme at the DBT service. Which *single* component is most likely found as part of this service? ★★

A Attention to group process

B Brief admission to hospital

C Interpretation of the transference

D Willingness to embrace Buddhist beliefs

E Weekly skills training group

11. A 16-year-old adolescent feels low in mood and lacks concentration at school. She says she has been unable to sleep at night since her parents' divorce six months ago. She is diagnosed with depression and referred for IPT. What is the *single* most appropriate description of this therapy? ★★

A It does not include homework inbetween sessions

B It is a therapy where therapeutic alliance is not relevant

C It is an open-ended treatment

D It is less effective than CBT in the treatment of depression

E The therapist uses direct questions to uncover hidden problems

12. A 29-year-old man has schizophrenia, with four admissions in the last six years due to a return of his symptoms. He stops taking his medication as soon as he is discharged from hospital. He comes from a close family but he says his family makes his illness worse. Family therapy is recommended and his father would like to know what the reasoning is for suggesting this intervention. Which is the *single* most appropriate answer to give? ★★★

A Compliance is improved

B It prevents other members of the family becoming delusional

C It stops family members becoming more critical of each other

D Overall cost of treatment is unchanged

E Relapses are spotted faster

13. A 36-year-old man has anticipatory anxieties. When he plans to go out for an evening run, he starts worrying about it from the morning. He worries about getting old, becoming ill, and having difficulties in his sexual life. His therapist helps him to discover his true end goals in life and how his current behaviours, emotions, or cognitions are impacting on those goals. From this manageable position subgoals are established and barriers to these are identified. Which is the *single* most likely behavioural therapy used? ★★★

A Acceptance and commitment therapy (ACT)

B Exposure and response prevention

C Functional analytic psychotherapy

D Habit reversal training

E Operant conditioning

14. A 56-year-old man suffers from flashbacks, difficulty in sleeping, and increased irritability following an RTC two months ago. He avoids going to the same area where the accident took place. Which is the *single* most appropriate treatment to recommend? ★★★

A Art therapy

B Counselling

C Eye movement desensitization and reprocessing

D Systemic therapy

E Watchful waiting

15. A 42-year-old woman with a diagnosis of emotionally unstable PD is admitted to the psychiatric ward following a significant overdose. During her stay on the ward, her relationship with staff deteriorates and she is reported as being a 'difficult and clingy patient' who staff avoid working with. She is provocative toward staff, telling them she is going to hurt herself and trying to arouse their anxiety through alarming statements such as 'I'll be dead by next year'. Which is the *single* most likely cause of her behaviour? ★★★

A Anankastic traits

B Malignant alienation

C Negative automatic thoughts

D Reciprocal roles

E Therapeutic alliance

16. A 23-year-old woman has superficial cuts on her arms and legs and scars from previous cuts dating back over seven years. She has been seen in the ED on several occasions having taken an overdose. She says that she has low self-esteem, body image problems, and significant difficulties in her relationships. She is referred to the specialist day hospital where they use mentalization-based therapy. Which is the *single* most appropriate description of this therapy? ★★★

A It demonstrates how to interpret all human behaviour in terms of intentional beliefs

B It focuses on patients' thoughts about themselves so they can understand others' reactions

C It helps patients examine their behaviour in order to promote healthy behaviour

D It places patients in challenging situations to help them learn to avoid them in the future

E It promotes reality testing activities to differentiate between truth and misperception

17. A 36-year-old woman suffers from intense feelings of rejection, low self-worth, and dependency on other people. During her psychodynamic psychotherapy session, she feels angry and upset that the therapist is going to be on leave the following week. She shows her anger by not attending the two consecutive sessions after the therapist comes back from leave. Which *single* defence mechanism most appropriately describes the patient's behaviour? ★★★

A Acting out
B Dissociation
C Projection
D Repression
E Undoing

18. A 28-year-old woman tells her therapist that she believes that she has to be perfect in everything she does and she cannot allow herself to make any mistakes. During her treatment, it came to light that she has internalized her parents' demands for her as a young girl to be 'the best in everything she did'. The therapist believes that Freud's structural theory is very relevant to this patient's experience. Which is the *single* most likely part of this theoretical model to be involved? ★★★★

A Ego
B Id
C Preconscious
D Superego
E Unconscious

19. A 38-year-old woman takes an overdose following a break-up with her partner. She says she has been unhappy for the last ten months and has little motivation to get a job, clear her debt, and make contact with her friends. Following discharge from the hospital, she is referred for cognitive analytic therapy (CAT). She would like to know what the aims of the therapist are during treatment. Which is the *single* most accurate description to give her? ★★★★

A Discussing problems within the patient rather than between the patient and others

B Focusing on mentalizing deficits in the patient's repertoire

C Identifying chains of events, thoughts, and emotions that maintain the problem

D Teaching mindfulness techniques to help the patient to regulate her emotions

E Waiting for the patient to bring up her difficulties without asking leading questions

20. A 22-year-old new mother is very low in mood and anxious that her four-month-old baby is not feeding well. She thinks the baby is crying excessively because he does not like her and she is not a good enough parent. Her GP refers her to local services for parent–infant psychotherapy. She asks what this involves. Which is the *single* most appropriate answer to give? ★★★★

A Fathers are excluded from the treatment plan

B It will focus on the temperament of the baby

C Sessions will include the mother and therapist alone

D The aim is to promote the parent–infant relationship

E Therapy has no planned end date

Extended Matching Questions

Types of therapy

For each description below, choose the *single* most appropriate talking therapy from the list of options. Each option may be used once, more than once, or not at all. ★★

A CBT

B Counselling

C DBT

D Eye movement desensitization and reprocessing

E Hypnotherapy

F IPT

G Mentalization-based treatment

H Problem-solving approach

I Psychodynamic psychotherapy

J Supportive therapy

1. A 34-year-old man is in therapy because he has difficulties in managing relationships. During treatment the therapist identifies four general areas in which he may have relationship difficulties: grief, conflict, difficulties adapting to changes, and social isolation.

2. A 45-year-old man has low mood, sleep difficulties, and low self-esteem. During treatment, the therapist helps him to recognize his core beliefs and consider negative automatic thoughts.

3. A 32-year-old woman is unable to use public transport due to excessive worry that people will look at her and will start talking about her. As part of her treatment, the therapist uses a session to ride with the patient on a bus and consider what takes place.

4. A 42-year-old woman feels rejected and criticized in all her relationships. During her therapy, the therapist makes use of unconscious redirection of feelings from the patient to the therapist to understand the patient's problems.

5. A 23-year-old woman has been self-harming by superficially cutting her forearm since the age of 16. She has low mood, low self-esteem, and significant relationship problems. As part of her treatment her therapist teaches her meditation techniques and focuses on her emotional regulation.

Cognitive distortion

For each description below, choose the single most appropriate type of cognitive distortion from the list of options. Each option may be used once, more than once, or not at all. ★★

A All or nothing thinking

B Arbitrary inference

C Compensatory misconceptions

D Disqualifying the positive

E Emotional reasoning

F Fortune telling

G Magnification/minimization

H Overgeneralization

I Personalization

J Selective abstraction

6. A 49-year-old woman receives CBT to treat her depression. She says that her PhD in molecular science was not worth anything and anybody can do it.

7. A 16-year-old adolescent who is preparing for exams, experiences excessive anxiety and inability to concentrate and sleep at night. She says to her therapist that if she gets any Bs, her whole life will be over, she will not be accepted to university, and she will not get any good jobs in the future.

8. A 25-year-old woman who experiences low self-esteem tells her therapist that her boyfriend did not call her that morning. She thinks it must because she must have said something wrong to him and now he probably hates her and will break up with her tonight.

9. A 59-year-old man has low mood. He tells his therapist that he saw his daughter over the weekend. He says that she 'does not think much of me' and has never taken him seriously because he feels undermined by her behaviour.

10. A 55-year-old woman who has generalized anxiety says in her therapy session that she was feeling upset the previous evening. She says that she was late to a dinner party and caused her friend to overcook the meal. She says if she had only pushed her partner to leave on time, it wouldn't have happened.

ANSWERS

Single Best Answers

1. A ★   OHPsych 3rd edn → pp.252–3

Psychological treatments are an important therapeutic option for people with depression. CBT is recommended as one of the first-line treatments for depression according to NICE guidelines (A). CBT can be delivered to individual patients or to a group. It requires active involvement of the patient. It is time limited and is focused on the here-and-now. The patient meets with a therapist for between five and 20 weekly or fortnightly sessions. Each session will last between 30 and 60 minutes. With the help of the therapist, the patient identifies individual patterns of thoughts, emotions, bodily sensations, and actions. Together they will work out if they are unrealistic or unhelpful and how they affect each other. The therapist will then help the patient to work out how to change unhelpful thoughts and behaviours. According to NICE guidelines, CBT has the best evidence base for efficacy, but it is not effective for everyone. The availability of alternatives drawing from a different theoretical model is therefore also important. However, it should be considered as a first-line treatment here.

Dance movement therapy (B) is the psychotherapeutic use of movement and dance through which a person can engage creatively in a process to further their emotional, cognitive, physical, and social integration. It tends to be used to help with stress and anxiety, particularly in patients with chronic diseases, for example cancer.

Music therapy (C) uses sound and music as a therapeutic medium to bring about change. According to the British Association for Music Therapy, it is effective in 'many clinical situations, particularly where communication is difficult due to illness, injury or disability'.

Play therapy (D) helps children understand muddled feelings and upsetting events by using play to communicate at their own level and at their own pace, without feeling interrogated or threatened.

Psychodrama (E) employs guided dramatic action to examine problems or issues raised by an individual using experiential methods, sociometry, role theory, and group dynamics. It can be used in affective disorders, especially in drug-resistant depression, but not as a first-line treatment.

→ NICE Clinical Guideline 90/91—Quick reference guide: Depression: http://www.nice.org.uk/nicemedia/pdf/CG%2090%20 QRG%20LR%20FINAL.pdf.

2. D ★   OHPsych 3rd edn → pp.404–5

Family therapy (D) is the recommended psychological treatment for anorexia nervosa in adolescents. The family are used to support the young person in their eating and consider why the eating disorder arose.

When the patient begins to accept the demand for increased food intake and steady weight gain, the driving force is often the family. Parents aim to work together to help their child take more control over their eating. In many cases, once the 'eating disorder' is no longer so dangerous, there are other general family relationship issues that need to be managed, such as day-to-day adolescent or parenting concerns. These are normal worries which the family has been forced to postpone due to the anorexia but which now start to arise. Family therapy can help with these too.

Attachment-based (psycho) therapy (A) is based on attachment theory. It is much like psychoanalysis targeted at problematic attachment styles which seeks to identify and challenge behaviours based on these misaligned attachments. Attachment styles include secure, anxious, avoidant, ambivalent, and disorganized attachments, some of which are thought to lead to later life difficulties. No direct correlation has been made with anorexia and this is not yet considered a first-line treatment option.

CBT is not the most appropriate psychological treatment to recommend (B). There are some who argue that there is limited efficacy of using talking therapies while the young person is underweight as there are known cognitive deficits at low BMI, which resolve when weight is gained. They advocate using a strict behavioural therapy regime which increases weight without tackling the emotional and psychology factors driving the weight loss. This is not, however, the recommended NICE guideline or a first-line treatment as it often results in an immediate return to the anorexic thinking and behaviours once the behavioural therapy is stopped.

DBT (C) is a form of therapy that is more appropriate in a patient with an emerging, or emerged, PD. While there is self-harming behaviour in anorexia, it tends to be chronic and focused on neglect/harm through not eating rather than the impulsive actions demonstrated in these cases. For patients with a PD emotions can be overwhelming and need immediate support.

Psychodynamic psychotherapy (E) may be of some use to the individual, but it will not help the family as a whole manage the situation or support them in helping the individual manage their eating behaviours. It would be something to consider at a later date once the eating is under control.

→ Eisler I, Dare C, Russell GFM, Szmukler G, le Grange D, Dodge E (1997). Family and individual therapy in anorexia nervosa: a 5-year follow-up. *Archives of General Psychiatry*, **54** (11), 1025–30.

→ NICE Clinical Guideline 9—Quick reference guide: Eating disorders: http://www.nice.org.uk/nicemedia/live/10932/29217/29217. pdf.

3. E ★　　　　OHPsych 3rd edn → pp.842–3.

Although the term 'mistake' is probably not used, the aim of group work is partly to allow group members to gain insight into their own problems by listening to the experiences of others and noticing the causes of their maladaptive behaviour and the subsequent difficulties produced (E). It is often easier to spot these issues in other people and it is not a cliché to say that people can often learn better from the mistakes of others. By seeing these issues arise, it can help a person to gain insight into their own problems and how to manage them.

Competition (A) is not encouraged as the group should work cooperatively rather than against each other. In a group where there are members at different stages of recovery, a member can be inspired by another member who has overcome a problem with which they are still struggling, rather than feel that they are losing against them.

Confidentiality (B) is still of the utmost importance. During group work members will share sensitive information and discuss matters of emotional and personal resonance, and they should feel confident that these discussions will not be shared with people outside the group (unless there is a clinical reason to do so). Normally groups will set out ground rules at the start of each session or period, which will include confidentiality as well as courtesy rules such as arriving on time and turning off mobile phones.

The point of this work is to discuss and share problems with progress rather than hide them away (C). By doing this, other group members can offer their own insight into why things are problematic and what could be done to help. Nobody wants to hear stories of misfortune, but to pretend they didn't happen would give false hope and only delay solving them.

While silence is not encouraged, it is not punished or highlighted (D). To do this would cause some members to disengage entirely and set back their treatment. Groups work best when everyone is involved, but some members, particularly at the early stages, may not have the confidence to talk. These members can still contribute to the group through non-verbal supportive behaviour, for example nodding, and in turn they will observe 'good' group behaviours being modelled by others.

---

4. E ★   OHPsych 3rd edn → pp.828–9

Using these feelings as a tool to understand the patient is the most appropriate response (E). Countertransference is the thoughts and feelings of the therapist in response to the patient's unconscious transference communications. In this example, he feels good because he has been told that he is 'special'. It is important to consider these thoughts and feelings when thinking about the patient, for example, they are a useful guide to the patient's expectations of relationships and worth remembering should she become upset or angry later on.

Although these feelings may be considered inappropriate, or just wrong, it would not be therapeutic to challenge them directly or expect the patient to be able to interpret them at that time (A). She may genuinely believe them to be correct when she says them and cannot see that they are part of a dangerous pattern in her relationships.

While it is nice to be praised and it takes practice to not feel good when given a compliment, it is worth remembering to reflect on the meaning behind the words and the driving forces leading her to believe these words to be true (B).

Keeping these statements confidential from the MDT (C) is not an appropriate response. The MDT acts to clarify the actions and thoughts of patients and therapists through team discussion and interpretation. This is a vital role in ongoing therapy. While gossip or non-clinically relevant parts of the work should not be brought to the team, these countertransference reactions should. At the start of a piece of work, a clear explanation should take be given about the role of the MDT and confidentiality.

Refusing to see a patient (D) based on a voicing of their emotions and feelings is a dangerous message to send. They may feel abandoned, rejected, and angry and might act impulsively to punish themselves or the therapist. It would be better to demonstrate that the therapist has a healthy ability to act not only within boundaries but also with a caring manner whether they are praised or criticized and that they will not be 'scared off'. Obviously, this may need to be rethought through should the patient become overly attached, for example asking the therapist on a date or attempting to form a sexual relationship with the therapist.

→ Hughes P, Kerr I (2000). Transference and countertransference in communication between doctor and patient. *Advances in Psychiatric Treatment*, **6**, 57–64.

5. D ★   OHPsych 3rd edn → pp.830–1

The answer is splitting (D). This is defined as a state where a person is seen as either good ('perfect') or bad ('evil'). The doctor is good and the nurse is bad. The patient treats them this way which in turn influences them to unconsciously play this out in their work relationship.

Idealization (A) is the act of attributing excessively positive qualities to someone else (or yourself). Although the patient is doing this it is only half the situation. She is enacting devaluation on the nurse, with wholly negative qualities.

Projective identification (B) is the act of projecting negative emotions onto another person and then attacking them. A man dislikes his boss because he reminds him of his father (who mistreated him), so he begins to act unkindly toward him, thereby annoying the boss, who then begins to treat him unfairly.

Rationalization (C) occurs where a person is certain that there was nothing wrong and that the difficulties are due to mistakes. Excuses are made even if they are tenuous. Here the patient does not make excuses but is ignoring the reality of the situation.

The mature defence mechanism of sublimation (E) is being demonstrated by the person performing other, usually more worthwhile, activities. For example, the young child who enjoys cutting up animals becomes a surgeon.

→ Winston AP (2000). Recent developments in borderline personality disorder. *Advances in Psychiatric Treatment*, **6**, 211–17.

6. C ★★ OHPsych 3rd edn → pp.840–1

Individual psychodynamic psychotherapy is an explorative psychotherapy which relies on the interpersonal relationship between therapist and patient more than other forms of depth psychology. Patients are encouraged to talk about their thoughts and feelings, including the ones they have about the therapy and the therapist (C). The patient's defences are thought about and are worked through to provide an understanding of the difficulties.

No official tasks or homework are given at the end of the session (A). However, there is an expectation that the themes and emotions raised in the session will remain in the patient's conscious and subconscious mind and be thought about after the session is over.

Unlike CBT or some of the more structured forms of talking therapy, psychodynamic psychotherapy can last for years. With this in mind it is worth considering how much time the patient has to spare on their treatment and what commitment they are willing to make. This is not considered to be a 'quick fix' therapy (B).

Sessions tend to be consistent throughout in as many ways as possible, including length, timing, location, and room layout. The idea is to avoid distractions such as sessions finishing unexpectedly or creating feelings of abandonment by being told that the session is shorter than usual (D). On occasions, patients may act to (unconsciously) push the boundaries of the therapist by bringing up controversial topics toward the end of the session in an effort to see if the therapist will still end the sessions as planned. The advice is that they should, but to pick up on the act and its implications at the next session.

The image of the psychotherapist on a seat behind a patient lying on a couch is widely held (E). It stems from Sigmund Freud, the father of psychoanalysis, who popularized psychotherapy. It was thought that he did this to avoid eye contact or possibly to avoid distracting the patient with his reactions. In modern psychotherapy, the therapist is just as likely to sit opposite the patient (who is also sitting) in the same manner as in a clinic.

→ Holmes J (1994). Brief dynamic psychotherapy. *Advances in Psychiatric Treatment*, **1**, 9–25.

→ Hook J (2001). The role of psychodynamic psychotherapy in a modern general psychiatry service. *Advances in Psychiatric Treatment*, **7**, 461–8.

7. D ★★ OHPsych 3rd edn → pp.376–8

The patient suffers from obsessive compulsive disorder. The mostly widely practised behaviour therapy for this is exposure and response prevention which is a CBT technique. The 'exposure' part of this treatment involves controlled exposure to objects or situations that arouse anxiety. Before starting, a hierarchical list of stimuli which the patient is worried about is produced (D), ranking the stimuli from most anxiety provoking to least anxiety provoking. The exposure is initially with the least anxiety provoking, before the patient moves up the list. Over time, exposure to obsessional cues leads to less and less anxiety. During treatment, patients learn to resist the compulsion to perform rituals and are eventually able to stop engaging in these behaviours.

Although childhood experiences may have helped shaped the worries, they are not the focus of this type of therapy (A). Instead the work is about the here-and-now of how the anxiety is provoked and then reduced. Its origins are not considered.

Experiments can be a mix of real or imaginary situations, and thus (B) is not the correct answer. If, for example, the worry is about spiders, then the most anxiety-provoking stimuli would be a real spider to hold, but even imagining a spider will cause a rise in stress hormones and may precipitate panic. Starting with imagined experiments can allow the patient to gain a mastery of their reactions in these situations first before attempting more difficult ones.

Any experiment in this therapy should provoke anxiety, otherwise it is not challenging the patient to acknowledge and manage their reaction to this. However, they may work to observe the anxiety start to fall or reduce to a manageable level rather than disappear completely (C). It is OK for someone to feel a little worried about dirt as long as it does not prevent them from functioning.

The initial work is focused in the session, but at all times homework is given and there is an expectation that the sessions will be thought about, planned, and worked on outside of the session. The therapist may put a limit on what should be attempted outside the session to avoid the patient becoming overwhelmed and feeling as though they 'failed' the experiment (E). As with any training, the focus is on a steady increase in ability rather than rushing to achieve each new thing.

→ Veale D (2007). Cognitive-behavioural therapy for obsessive-compulsive disorder. *Advances in Psychiatric Treatment*, **13**, 438–46.

8. E ★★   OHPsych 3rd edn → pp.250–1

Severe depression is best treated with antidepressant medication. In this case, an SSRI would be the most suitable first-line treatment (E). There is a high incidence of depression in cancer that is thought to be due to the diagnosis itself but also to the symptoms of the cancer, for example loss of sexual function and incontinence in prostate cancer. There have been some reported associations between antidepressant drug use, particularly older antidepressants, and the risk of cancer, but SSRIs were not found to be significantly associated with the risk of prostate cancer.

CBT (A) can be effective in treating depression in terminal illness. However, this man has a severe depression which would respond better in the first instance to medication rather than a talking therapy. It is important to consider the evidence base for any intervention in the context of the most pressing problem—in this case severe depression. After establishing him on an antidepressant it would be sensible to consider combining a psychotherapeutic approach.

Gestalt therapy (B) is generally used where there are difficulties caused by a person's personality. It emphasizes self-reliance and acceptance. It focuses on one's own experience at the present moment, in both the clinical and social context, while seeking to highlight the self-regulating adjustments we make to manage difficult experiences. There is no evidence to suggest it would be beneficial here.

Grief counselling (C) has a place in working with patients who have been diagnosed with a terminal illness. It can help that person work through their emotions and gain acceptance of the situation. However, it is not effective where there is a severe mental illness such as depression. Grief counselling can be delivered by any trained counsellor, including healthcare professionals, religious leaders, and those in the voluntary sector.

Psychodynamic psychotherapy (D) can be used in patients with a terminal illness. However, there are as yet no published studies on the effectiveness of individual psychotherapy on recurrence or survival time. Psychodynamic therapy will most likely consider looking at the defences and coping mechanisms in place (considered to be an 'ego-led' model).

→ National Cancer Institute—Suicide Risk in Patients with Cancer: http://www.cancer.gov/cancertopics/pdq/supportivecare/depression/Patient/page4.

9. C ★★　　　OHPsych 3rd edn → pp.850–3

Negative automatic thoughts (C) most accurately describes this. They are ideas that are situation specific and pop into a person's mind when they are experiencing some kind of emotional distress.

Core beliefs (A) are absolute statements about the self, others, or the world and the future which were often learned in childhood and are treated as if they are absolute facts.

Mentalization (B) is the ability to understand the mental state of oneself and others which underlies overt behaviour.

Reciprocal roles (D) is a concept in CAT, but reciprocal thoughts is not a term used in psychiatry.

Underlying assumptions (E) are the patient's rules or values—that predispose them to depression, anxiety, or anger.

→ Beck A (1976). Cognitive therapy and the emotional disorders. Penguin, London.

10. E ★★　　　OHPsych 3rd edn → pp.856–7

The answer is a weekly skills training group (E). DBT combines standard CBT for emotion regulation and reality-testing with concepts of distress tolerance, acceptance, and mindful awareness. Components of DBT include individual sessions, a skills training group, out-of-hours telephone contact, and a consultation group.

While receiving DBT patients have individual work and group work which complement each other; the individual work aims to keep impulsive emotions and suicidal ideation from breaking up group work, while the group sessions focus on the skills unique to DBT. Group work provides a rehearsal place to regulate emotions, actions, and behaviours in a realistic context. Therefore attention to group process (A) is not the answer.

Neither is brief admission to hospital (B), as DBT works with patients who are living in the 'real world' rather than in the hospital setting. This does mean that a consideration must be taken whether an individual is of too high a risk to start DBT at that time.

Transference and its interpretation (C) is used in psychodynamic psychotherapy rather than in DBT. In DBT there is a move toward learning to bear psychological pain rather than focusing on changing distressing events and situations.

Although mindfulness practice is used in DBT, and it is inherited from the Buddhist tradition, patients using DBT don't have to follow the other beliefs of Buddhism (D). That said, the belief that 'nothing is fixed or permanent—change is always possible' is one that is reflected in much of psychiatry.

→ Palmer RL (2002). Dialectical behaviour therapy for borderline personality disorder. *Advances in Psychiatric Treatment*, **8**, 10–16.

11. A ★★   OHPsych 3rd edn → pp.854–5

In IPT, homework, such as behavioural experiments, is not given (A), which makes it particularly accessible to patients who find the dynamic approaches or the 'homework' demands of CBT difficult. However, even though effort isn't needed for homework tasks, IPT involves the re-enactment of past negative feelings, which, as well as creating a danger of emotional harm, requires more effort than is needed in CBT sessions. It is by no means an 'easy therapy'.

(B) is not the correct answer as the therapeutic relationship and collaboration between the therapist and the patient are very important. IPT avoids psychotherapy jargon in order to help facilitate this alliance. It has an exploratory rationale and aims to share understanding between the patient and the therapist. The fundamental clinical task of IPT is to help link mood with interpersonal relationships. By recognizing and appropriately addressing these issues patients improve their relationships and in turn lift their depressive state.

IPT is a time-limited therapy (not open-ended (C)) which is structured to last for 12–16 weeks. It focuses on relationships: the difficulty in starting relationships and keeping them going, especially due to interpersonal conflicts. It also considers how life changes affect how a person feels about themselves and others.

IPT is evidence-based psychotherapy. It has been evaluated as both an acute intervention and a maintenance therapy for major depression. It has been adapted for use across different age groups including adolescents and older people. IPT was originally designed as an individual therapy, but it has been modified for use in a group setting. Several studies have found little difference in the effectiveness between IPT and CBT (D). It has also been reported that patients expressed a preference for IPT over CBT, which would help to promote increased adherence.

The therapist uses statements rather than asking questions (E). It is important that the patient does not feel under the spotlight. The therapist helps the patient to link their symptoms to the interpersonal context and to clarify any emergent themes. Some sessions may open with general questions about events and experiences since the last meeting in order to focus on current, rather than historic, encounters.

→ Guthrie E (1999). Psychodynamic interpersonal therapy. *Advances in Psychiatric Treatment*, **5**, 135–45.

12. A ★★★   OHPsych 3rd edn → p.208

Family therapy in schizophrenia improves treatment compliance (A), reduces relapse rates, and reduces expressed emotions in the family.

The therapy in itself does not aim to stop any other family members from becoming unwell (B). Given the genetic link in schizophrenia there is already an increased likelihood of a first-degree relative having/developing a mental illness. However, the therapy should improve the family environment and reduce stress within the family, which may act to lessen the precipitating factors for developing a psychotic illness. The role of epigenetics in schizophrenia is not yet fully explained.

Family therapy allows the family to communicate in a safe environment, with a focus on healthy exploration of the family dynamics. This does not mean that everyone can *only* say nice, uncritical things to each other. In fact, sometimes things are said in the relative safety of the therapeutic environment that are more critical than the person would feel comfortable saying at home (C).

Although family therapy has an associated cost from the trained therapists involved and the facilities needed, the cost of an inpatient admission is much greater (D). If it can reduce relapse and allow for a return to work, etc. then the overall cost impact will be profitable.

Family therapists are trained and experienced in working with people with mental illness, but there is no guarantee that a relapse will be spotted any faster due to the therapy itself (E). It is clear that better compliance and a reduced expression of emotion in the family will reduced the number and frequency of relapses.

→ Leff J (1998). Needs of the families with people with schizophrenia. *Advances in Psychiatric Treatment*, **4**, 277–84.

13. A ★★★   OHPsych 3rd edn → pp.820–1, 845

ACT (A) is a form of behavioural analysis and the most likely therapy used. It mixes acceptance, mindfulness, and behaviour-change strategies, to increase 'psychological flexibility'. The therapist helps the patient understand that their current state might be because they are stuck in a problematic situation which they haven't been able to change. This is not because their problem-solving abilities are ineffectual, but because they are trying to solve the wrong problem. One of the major assumptions is that language is relational—that cognitions, emotions, and actions all need to be understood in context. The focus is on changing the context of the thoughts and emotions. The therapist helps the patient to discover his true end goals in life and how his current behaviours, emotions, or cognitions are (or are not) detracting from those goals.

Exposure and response prevention (B) is a behavioural therapy based on the theory that a positive therapeutic effect is achieved when patients repeatedly challenge themselves with specific anxiety-provoking situations and do not allow themselves to be overwhelmed by the anxiety. After doing this a number of times, the anxiety produced in these situations is reduced until it is manageable. The behavioural process is called 'Pavlovian extinction' and its background is in classical conditions where repeated exposure to an event without any subsequent reinforcement caused the reaction to diminish over time before disappearing entirely. In this case, the anxiety is derived more from general worry than a specific situation or thing, which would make this therapy less effective. Exposure and response prevention is primarily for anxiety disorders, such as phobia, and for the treatment of OCD.

Functional analytic psychotherapy (C) is a mixture of CBT and psychodynamic approaches which hopes to improve interpersonal relationships. It focuses on both behaviours and the driving forces behind those behaviours by offering psychoanalytical interpretations alongside behavioural analysis. In a session the patient presents their 'problem' and their verbal behaviour is considered using the therapeutic alliance and psychoanalytic (transference and countertransference) techniques. It is not, however, a recommended treatment at this time and currently lacks a wider acceptance in either branch of psychotherapy.

Habit reversal training (D) is a behavioural therapy used for damaging repetitive behaviours such as tics, nail biting, and skin picking. It has five components: awareness training (spotting where the behaviours take place and what happens), competing response training (doing something else instead of the harmful behaviour), motivation (getting others involved to help promote the new behaviours), relaxation training, and generalization training (practising these skills in new environments). It would not be helpful in this scenario due to the higher cognitive element of the anxiety.

Operant conditioning (E) was described by B.F. Skinner in 1937 as a method by which behaviours can be directly encouraged or discouraged through reward or punishment (or the withdrawal of either). It is used in various forms throughout psychology and has been adapted for use in groups and animals. At its core is the recognition that actions that are rewarded are repeated and those that are not rewarded, or punished, are not repeated. Operant conditioning can be used in young children, such as 'time outs', in institutions, using the token economies, or in the wider community, such as taxes. In this case, the anxieties are anticipatory in nature and not easily modulated through reward or 'punishment'.

→ Association for Contextual Behavioral Science:

http://contextualpsychology.org/about_act.

14. C ★★★ OHPsych 3rd edn → pp.392–3

The patient has PTSD. Trauma-focused CBT or eye movement desensitization and reprocessing (C) are recommended as the first-line treatments for

PTSD according to NICE guidelines. This is a form of therapy in which the patient recalls a traumatic event while simultaneously undergoing bilateral stimulation, which can consist of moving the eyes from side to side, vibrations or tapping movements on different sides of the body, or tones delivered through one ear, then the other, via headphones.

Art therapy (A) is a form of psychotherapy that uses art media as its primary mode of communication. Patients do not need to be skilful in art as the art therapist is. They are not making an aesthetic or diagnostic assessment of the image produced. The aim, according to the British Association of Art Therapists, is to 'enable a client to effect change and growth on a personal level through the use of art materials in a safe and facilitating environment'. There is no specific focus on the trauma and therefore this would not be a first-line treatment in this case.

Counselling (B) is a type of talking therapy where the patient discusses their feelings, difficulties, or emotions in a confidential and safe environment. While some counsellors may be trained to help people with PTSD, this should be established before the therapy starts and an agreement reached that this is the focus of the work. In many cases counselling is aimed at less acute conditions such as mild depression, anxiety, or long-term illness rather than PTSD.

NICE guidelines do not recommend non-trauma-focused interventions to be offered routinely if the patient presents within three months of trauma. It is not clear that the systemic therapy will be focused on the trauma (D).

There are clear symptoms of PTSD which are causing distress to the patient and a disruption to their life. There is no reason to expect that these will resolve without an intervention and therefore watchful waiting should not be suggested at this time (E).

→ MacCulloch MJ (1999). Eye movement desensitization and reprocessing. *Advances in Psychiatric Treatment*, **5**, 120–5.

→ NICE Clinical Guideline 26—Quick Reference Guide: Post-traumatic stress disorder: http://www.nice.org.uk/nicemedia/pdf/cg026quick-refguide.pdf.

| 15. **B** ★★★ | OHPsych 3rd edn → pp.508–9 |

Malignant alienation (B) is characterized by a progressive deterioration in a patient's relationship with others, including loss of sympathy and support from members of staff, who tended to construe these patients' behaviour as provocative, unreasonable, or overdependent. Patients involved in this process may have long-standing problems communicating their needs effectively. This results in them attempting to have their care needs met in less appropriate ways which are not effective or considered appropriate. Instead they provoke ambivalent or negative response in their carers. Malignant alienation was identified in 55% of suicides amongst inpatients in one study.

Anankastic traits (A) are seen most often as part of obsessional PD. People with these traits are sensitive to criticism, dependent on others, and often have unexpressed feelings of anger and resentment. The difficult behaviour is usually an unreasonable insistence by the patient that others submit to exactly their way of doing things, or unreasonable reluctance to allow others to do things in a different manner. They are not usually associated with overdoses, provocative behaviour, or upsetting staff.

Negative automatic thoughts (C) are negatively framed interpretations of what we think is happening to us. They are our own thoughts, rather than a psychotic phenomenon, which are usually accepted as reality without question, resulting in a destructive impact on mood and feelings. If unchallenged they can lead to self-doubt, irritability, and low mood. These are usually seen in depression and are the target of CBT. In this patient it is unlikely that her provocative statements are being driven by negative thoughts, although she may have unrealistic and damaging reactions to her own thoughts and emotions.

Reciprocal roles (D) are part of the work of Ryle and used in CAT. He described a theory that as children we learn about the social world and store behaviours as internalized templates of reciprocal roles. This includes how we see ourselves and others, and how relationships 'work'. They can be functional (e.g. caregiver/care receiver) or dysfunctional (abuser/abused). Later in life we act to take up one pole of a reciprocal-role pairing, and the other person is under pressure to adopt the congruent pole. If this patient has learnt that the world involves victims and bullies then they may act to place members of the MDT into these two roles and themselves in the opposite.

This is the relationship between any healthcare professional and patient. By engaging with each other in a positive manner, beneficial change is seen. It can also be seen between patients, relatives, colleagues, and any of the MDT. Part of this alliance is the 'working alliance' where the patient and therapist agree upon tasks to reach goals: what the patient hopes to gain from therapy, based on their presenting problems. The therapeutic alliance (E) is essential in establishing and maintaining confidence that the tasks will result in a positive outcome.

→ Watts D, Morgan G (1994). Malignant alienation. Dangers for patients who are hard to like. *British Journal of Psychiatry*, **164**, 11–15.

16. A ★★★ OHPsych 3rd edn → pp.506–7

The most appropriate description is one which demonstrates how to interpret all human behaviour in terms of intentional beliefs (A). Mentalization is a psychological concept that describes the ability to understand the mental state of oneself and others which underlies overt behaviour. Mentalization can be seen as a form of imaginative mental activity, which allows us to perceive and interpret human behaviour in terms of intentional mental states (e.g. needs, desires, feelings, beliefs, goals, purposes, and reasons). It is about understanding misunderstandings, considering ourselves in relation to other people, and considering other people's states of mind. It is the normal ability to ascribe intentions and meaning to human behaviour. It is about seeing ourselves from the outside and others from the inside. The focus is not solely on examining one's own behaviour or thought but also to consider other people.

Focusing on patient's thoughts about themselves so they can understand others' reactions (B) is more the realm of psychotherapy that mentalization. While thoughts about themselves are important, they are not the focus. There is no clear link that understanding our own thoughts allows us to understand others and why they behave differently from ourselves.

Patients' own behaviour is not examined (C), rather it is about understanding how other people behave and how we interact with them.

Instead of planning for a future of avoidance (D), there is a focus on tolerating and accepting the powerful emotions that arise when patients challenge their habits or expose themselves to upsetting situations. This is similar to OCD treatment where the aim is not to avoid challenging situations but to learn to cope with them should they arise.

Reality testing (E) is important in differentiating between an external reality and an inner imaginative world. Without this we cannot behave in a manner that exhibits an awareness of accepted norms and customs. Impairment of reality testing is indicative of a disturbance in mental functioning which may be part of early psychosis. Here the patient knows what is external and internal but cannot manage her feelings.

→ Fonagy P, Bateman A (2006). Mentalization-based treatment for borderline personality disorder: a practical guide. Oxford University Press, Oxford.

17. A ★★★   OHPsych 3rd edn → pp.830–1

The answer is acting out (A), performing an extreme behaviour in order to express thoughts or feelings the person feels incapable of otherwise expressing. Instead of saying, 'I'm angry with you', a person who acts out may instead miss the following session.

Dissociation (B) provides the capacity to detach from disturbing emotional states such as emotional numbing, depersonalization and derealization, amnesia, and identity fragmentation.

Projection (C) is the misattribution of a person's unacceptable and undesired thoughts, feelings, or impulses onto another person.

Repression (D) is the unconscious blocking of unacceptable thoughts, feelings, and impulses.

Undoing (E) is the attempt to take back an unconscious behaviour or thought that is unacceptable or hurtful.

→ Bateman A, Holmes J (1995). Introduction to Psychoanalysis: Contemporary Theory and Practice, pp.76–94. Routledge, London.

→ Bowins B (2004). Psychological defense mechanisms, a new perspective. American Journal of Psychoanalysis, **64** (1).

18. D ★★★★   OHPsych 3rd edn → pp.824–5; 828

The superego (D) is most likely to be involved. It describes conscience and ideals which are derived through the internalization of parental or other authority figures. The superego is involved in the experience of guilt, perfectionism, indecision, and preoccupation with right or wrong.

Freud first used the topographical model to describe the human mind. It consists of the preconscious, conscious, and unconscious. Freud later on developed the structural model which consists of ego (A), id, and superego. The ego is the organized, realistic part that mediates between the desires of the id and the superego.

The id (B) is the set of uncoordinated instinctual trends.

The conscious contains all thoughts and ideas that are immediately received by the mind. These thoughts may include a person's perception, emotion, and intellectual processes. The contents of the preconscious (C) are not obstructed by any form of repression and are therefore accessible to the conscious.

The unconscious (E) stores all memories and ideas that are observed without the person knowing it. The unconscious also holds a person's desires, wishes, dreams, and fears.

→ Schafer R (1960). The loving and beloved superego in Freud's structural theory. In: Solnit AJ, Eissler RS, Freud A, Kris M, Neubauer PB (eds) *The Psychoanalytic Study of the Child*. International Universities Press, New York.

---

19. C ★★★★ OHPsych 3rd edn → pp.858–9

Identifying chains of events, thoughts, and emotions which maintain the problem (C) is the most accurate description. CAT is a collaborative therapy for looking at the way a person thinks, feels, and acts, and the events and relationships that underlie these experiences (often from childhood or earlier in life). It is a time-limited therapy—between 4 and 24 weeks, but typically 16. The model emphasizes collaborative work with the patient, and focuses on the understanding of the patterns of maladaptive behaviours. The aim of the therapy is to enable the patient to recognize these patterns, understand their origins, and subsequently to learn alternative coping strategies.

The focus is to identify problems as occurring between people and not just within the patient (A). This therapy acknowledges the importance of relationships in the patient's psychological life, including the relationship the patient has with him or herself as well as others. These patterns of relationship, called reciprocal roles, and how these patterns have been developed and what they produce will often be shown in the relationship between the client and the therapist.

Mentalization deficits (B) are worked through in mentalization-based treatment.

Mindfulness techniques (D) are used in DBT.

Waiting for the patient to bring up her difficulties without asking leading questions (E) is not the correct answer. In the first quarter of the therapy the therapist collects all the relevant information, asking the patient about present-day problems and also earlier life experiences. This involves leading questions and directive questions. After this they work together to construct a diagrammatic formulation of the patterns to illustrate the unhelpful procedures that maintain problems for the patient. This enables the patient to recognize when and how problems occur. Next the patient works to identify and practise 'exits' from the pattern. At the end of the therapy, patient and therapist each write 'goodbye letters' to summarize what has been achieved in the therapy and what remains to be done. There is usually a follow-up session after one month, then three months later.

→ Denman C (2001). Cognitive analytic therapy. *Advances in Psychiatric Treatment*, **7**, 243–52.

20. **D** ★★★★   OHPsych 3rd edn → pp. 820–1

Parent–infant psychotherapy is a relationship-based intervention that promotes the parent–infant relationship in order to facilitate infant development (D). The infant is the product of the continuous dynamic interaction of the infant, his or her family, and the social context.

All primary caregivers should be considered when planning the treatment. This will include the father (A), same sex partners, step-parents, etc. However, this differs from family therapy in that not everyone from the household will be automatically invited.

The infant is not independent of his or her environment. So, while temperament is important (B), the environment plays a significant part in determining the infant's experience as well as that of the parents. How the child develops cannot be considered without analysing both temperament and environment.

The therapy session includes both the parent(s) and the baby, not just the adults (C). It is important for the therapist to consider the interactions that take place within the parental unit, including those that are unconscious and non-verbal.

While there are not a limited number of sessions planned, as there is in CBT, there is usually an aim to finish within one year of starting the therapy (E). In every case, endings are planned for when parents and therapist consider there is sufficient improvement.

→ Baradon T (2005). *The Practice of Parent–Infant Psychoanalytical Psychotherapy*. Routledge, London.

Extended Matching Questions

1. F ★★

The therapist uses IPT techniques. IPT is a time-limited psychotherapy, usually six to twenty sessions, which focuses on relationships. These are thought to be responsible for precipitation and perpetuating psychological distress. It aims to improve interpersonal functioning and social support.

2. A ★★

The patient is suffering from depression. The treatment of choice is CBT. In depression, people get negative automatic thoughts which result in a misinterpretation of normal events to reinforce the low mood or difficult relationships. Evaluation of an event is decided by quick, instantaneous thoughts concerning the event. These thoughts emerge unconsciously and are accepted as true. Beck believed they originated from 'core beliefs' which were developed in childhood and never questioned or considered even if they were damaging.

3. A ★★

The patient suffers from social phobia, for which the first-time treatment is CBT. The experiment here is part of a wider plan to consider the particular worries the patient has and how realistic they are. These experiments help both the therapist and the patient test the validity of these beliefs and then to develop new beliefs, which can in turn be tested. For example, the patient may believe that everyone on the bus is looking at them, but having completed the experiment they may reconsider and decide that people are looking at them but also at other people and not in a judgemental manner.

4. I ★★

The therapist uses transference dynamics, which was explained by Freud as an unconscious redirection of feelings from one person to another, usually from a childhood experience. For example, if the patient feels that they were mistreated by a parent as a child, they can transfer their anger (and other emotions) onto the therapist, who in turn acts as a 'parent' in that relationship. Countertransference is the redirection of the therapist's feelings toward the patient. Both can lead to emotional entanglement if not dealt with appropriately.

5. C ★★

The 'meditation techniques' are also called mindfulness. This is one of the most important parts of DBT. It is thought to help by allowing the person to concentrate on the here-and-now experience while focusing their energy and attention in a regulated healthy manner. This allows for increased control over impulsive thoughts and actions when they arise.

→ General feedback on 1–5: OHPsych 3rd edn pp.820–3

→ Palmer RL (2002). Dialectical behaviour therapy for borderline personality disorder. *Advances in Psychiatric Treatment*, **8**, 10–16.

→ RCPsych information on psychotherapies: http://www.rcpsych.ac.uk/expertadvice/treatmentswellbeing/psychotherapies.aspx.

6. G ★★

When magnifying or minimizing, the patient exaggerates the importance of things or inappropriately shrinks things until they appear tiny. This is also called the 'binocular trick'. Normally the person will both shirk the positive aspects and maximize the negative ones, to create an even larger difference between the two and feel even worse.

7. A ★★

In all or nothing thinking, the patient sees things in black and white categories as opposed to shades of grey. In this way everything becomes split into something that will or won't happen, which results in wrong assumptions or unrealistic dilemmas. Often this type of splitting will result in using words like 'always', 'every', or 'never', which leave no room for subtlety.

8. F ★★

Fortune telling is a distortion where the patient makes a negative interpretation even though there are no definite facts that convincingly support her conclusion. In this way she is jumping to conclusions based on very little evidence and then predicting future events with a certainty that isn't warranted. This can be confused with catastrophization; however, for this to be the case there would need to be an actual event to take place (which could then be catastrophized), rather than the assumption of the event.

9. E ★★

Emotional reasoning is a distortion where the patient assumes that the way they feel reflects the reality of the way things are. In this way they believe that their feeling has exposed the true nature of things. For example, a person with a lot of revision to do can be overwhelmed by the prospect of the work and feel it's hopeless to do the work and therefore they do nothing as believe it won't lead to anything. In reality, it may feel hopeless but it rarely is.

10. I ★★

Personalization is a distortion where a person believes that everything others do or say is some kind of direct, personal reaction to the person. Thereby they assume that they take personal responsibility for the action and reaction and feel guilty for this.

General feedback on 6–10: OHPsych 3rd edn → pp.850–1

→ Hawton K, Salkovskis PM, Kirk J, Clark DM (1989). *Cognitive Behaviour Therapy for Psychiatric Problems: A Practical Guide*. Oxford Medical Publications, Oxford.

Chapter 8

Mental health and the law

Paula Murphy and Tim Exworthy

Mental health law is concerned with the legislation governing the management and treatment of people with a mental disorder. It includes the detention and treatment of patients and covers consent to treatment, mental capacity, deprivation of liberty, human rights, and ethical issues. The law is necessary to safeguard the interests of the patients and also to protect the public from potentially serious harm from a mentally disordered offender. It is crucial that mental health practitioners understand the relevant legislation to ensure that they are practising within the realms of the law and also so that they can offer help and advice to patients and carers if required to do so.

Mental health legislation is constantly evolving and there are always challenges and changes to existing legislation, so practitioners need to keep up to date with new statutory legislation and case law. An example of this is the Mental Health Act (MHA) 1983, which was amended by the MHA 2007, and amended again by the Health and Social Care Act 2012. In addition, the Mental Capacity Act 2005 was a new statute which came into force in 2007, alongside Deprivation of Liberty Safeguards.

There are Codes of Practice for the MHA, the Mental Capacity Act, and the Deprivation of Liberty Safeguards. These provide supplementary guidance on good practice. Mental health practitioners need to take account of the Codes of Practice in their work.

Mental health law can be a complex and challenging area, even for the most knowledgeable and experienced practitioners. Most organizations will have an MHA administrator and/or a legal advisor who can provide advice and guidance in matters of uncertainty.

Paula Murphy and Tim Exworthy

QUESTIONS

Single Best Answers

1. A 59-year-old woman with early-onset dementia is admitted to the ward. Her family are concerned that she has not written a will and appoint a solicitor for her. The solicitor would like to know about her ability to write a will. Which is the *single* most appropriate answer to give? ★

A Advise she does not have capacity

B Ask her nearest relative (NR) to assist in writing a will

C Ask the approved mental health professional to assist in writing a will

D Assess her mental capacity

E Assess her testamentary capacity

2. A 41-year-old man, who is detained on a section 3 of the MHA, would like to find out who has the power to discharge him from his section. Which is the *single* most appropriate answer to give? ★

A GP

B MHA managers

C Medical director

D Next of kin

E Ward doctor

3. A 39-year-old woman with paranoid schizophrenia and HIV is detained in hospital on a section 3 of the MHA. She is refusing all of her medications including her antiretroviral medications. She does not want active treatment for HIV. Which is the *single* most appropriate immediate course of action to take? ★

A Give antipsychotic medication under the MHA

B Give antiretroviral medication covertly

C Give antiretroviral medication under the MHA

D Give both medications covertly

E Give both medications under the MHA

4. A 36-year-old man is in a methadone maintenance programme. He works as a bus driver and has been told by the clinic in person and in writing that he must inform the DVLA that he is on methadone and that this disclosure is a legal requirement. He has refused to do so because of his job. Which is the *single* most appropriate initial action to take? ★

A Anonymously inform the DVLA

B Inform the patient's employer

C Inform the police

D Stop the methadone prescription

E Tell the patient that you are going to inform the DVLA

5. A 35-year-old man with schizophrenia discloses that he is having thoughts of killing his ex-girlfriend because he has found out that she has a new partner. When asked if he has any specific plan to do this he replies that he cannot say any more. He asks for this information to be kept confidential and for it not to be recorded in the notes. Which is the *single* most appropriate initial management? ★★

A Ask his permission to inform the police

B Document his disclosure in the notes as third party information

C Do not document his disclosure to keep it confidential

D Inform the patient's NR

E Inform the police without discussion

6. A 27-year-old man is currently an informal patient on the ward. He believes the nursing staff are controlling him through the computer and has smashed the window of the nursing station. De-escalation techniques have been unsuccessful and he is refusing oral medication. Nursing staff would like to administer rapid tranquillization. Which is the *single* most appropriate immediate course of action? ★★

A Advise watchful waiting to see if he calms down

B Organize an MHA assessment

C Rapid tranquillization under common law

D Rapid tranquillization under the Mental Capacity Act

E Rapid tranquillization using section 62 of the MHA

7. A 45-year-old man with BPAD is acutely manic when seen in the outpatient clinic. He is posing as a risk to himself and others. He refuses informal hospital admission. There is only one doctor available but there is an approved mental health professional on site. Which is the *single* most appropriate section of the MHA to use? ★★

A Section 2

B Section 3

C Section 4

D Section 5(2)

E Section 5(4)

8. A 31-year-old man with a history of schizophrenia was admitted two days ago on a section 3 of the MHA. He requires treatment with antipsychotic medication but has refused to take this orally. Which is the *single* most appropriate management? ★★

A Administer oral antipsychotic covertly

B Apply for a second-opinion approved doctor to assess for IM antipsychotic

C Prescribe IM antipsychotic for immediate use

D Prescribe IM antipsychotic under section 62 of the MHA

E Wait until he agrees to take oral medications

9. A 37-year-old woman made an advance decision when she had capacity against having ECT in the future. She is now severely depressed and is not responding to antidepressant medication. She does not have the capacity to consent to treatment currently. Which is the *single* most appropriate treatment to initiate? ★★★★

A Add lithium as an adjunct to her antidepressant mediation

B Apply for a second-opinion approved doctor to assess for ECT

C Give ECT as it is in her best interests

D Give ECT using a section 62 of the MHA

E Give ECT with consent of her NR

10. A 40-year-old man with a history of depression is assessed under the MHA by two doctors and an approved mental health professional. He is considered to require detention under the MHA on a section 3 for treatment that is necessary for his own health and safety, but his NR objects. Which is the *single* most appropriate management? ★★★★

A Apply to the Court to displace the NR

B Apply to the hospital manager to displace the NR

C Detain him against the wishes of the NR

D Do not detain him and arrange community follow-up

E Identify someone else as the NR

Extended Matching Questions

Sections of the MHA

For each scenario below, choose the *single* most appropriate section of the MHA to be used from the list of options. Each option may be used once, more than once, or not at all. ★★

A Section 2

B Section 3

C Section 5(2)

D Section 5(4)

E Section 36

F Section 37

G Section 47

H Section 48

I Section 135

J Section 136

1. A 35-year-old man is found by the police on the streets acting bizarrely and talking to himself. He believes that a microchip has been inserted in his head to monitor him. The police feel that he needs to be assessed by the emergency mental health services.

2. A 20-year-old woman on an obstetric ward had an emergency caesarean section one week ago. The midwives are concerned that the woman is not interacting with the baby and neglecting to feed her. She believes the baby is actually an imposter and not her real baby. She wants to leave hospital with the baby, but the duty doctor believes this would be unsafe.

3. A 48-year-old man who is serving a life sentence for murder is assessed in prison by the prison doctor. He has stopped eating because he believes the food has been poisoned by the prison staff. He hears voices telling him not to trust anyone. He is very guarded and is isolating himself. The prison doctor feels he needs to be transferred to hospital.

4. A 30-year-old man with a history of schizophrenia has been convicted for arson. He was acutely psychotic at the time of the offence. Psychiatric reports were requested by the Court to advise on disposal. Based on the psychiatric reports and recommendations, the Court decides to divert him to hospital rather than serve him with a prison sentence.

5. A 31-year-old woman is being assessed at home under the MHA. She is not attending to her personal care. She is withdrawn and vague and describes clear suicidal ideation. She has lost 12 kg over the last six weeks. It is decided that she requires further assessment in hospital. She is not known to psychiatric services.

Legal provisions

For each scenario below, choose the *single* most appropriate legal provision to consider from the list of options. Each option may be used once, more than once, or not at all. ★★★★

A Lasting Power of Attorney

B Deprivation of Liberty Safeguards

C Common law

D Community Treatment Order

E Guardianship Order

F Mental Capacity Act

G MHA

H No legal provisions apply

I Section 17 of the MHA

J Section 117 of the MHA

6. A 23-year-old man with alcohol dependency is brought to the ED by his mother who wants him to be detained under the MHA so that he can undergo alcohol detoxification and be treated for his addiction. The man does not want to be admitted to hospital.

7. A 35-year-old woman with learning disability is brought to the ED by her carers. Over the last few weeks she has become increasingly agitated and aggressive, and is now attacking staff and residents in her care home. The carers are finding it difficult to cope with her and want her to be admitted to hospital for assessment. The woman is incapable of consenting to admission but is not resisting it.

8. A 45-year-old man is convicted for a number of indecent sexual assaults against children. The Court has asked for a psychiatric assessment to assist with sentencing.

9. A 17-year-old woman with autism is no longer able to be cared for at home by her elderly parents. They are requesting a respite hospital admission until an appropriate residential home can be found for her. She is not capable of consenting.

10. A 30-year-old woman with emotionally unstable PD is seen in the ED following an overdose. She is medically cleared but is disappointed about her failed suicide attempt. She would like to leave hospital.

ANSWERS

Single Best Answers

1. E ★   OHPsych 3rd edn → pp.794–5

The most appropriate answer is to assess her testamentary capacity (E), i.e. her capacity to write a will. This is based on the testator being aware of: (1) what a will is and what its consequences are; (2) the nature and extent of his or her property; and (3) the names of close relatives and beneficiaries; moreover, they must be able to assess the latter's claims to his/her property. Additionally, the testator must not be acting on delusional ideas or be in such an emotional state that this might distort feelings or judgements relevant to making the will.

Adults over 18 years old must be assumed to have capacity unless it is established that they lack capacity. As this woman has dementia, an assessment is required to determine whether she has capacity to make a will. Capacity is decision specific, i.e. people may have capacity to make some decisions but not others (e.g. what to have for lunch, but not to decide where they will live). A person is not to be treated as unable to make a decision merely because they make an unwise decision (A).

Only the testator can write a will, so a relative cannot do this on her behalf (B). If the testator is not deemed to have capacity to write their own will then an application can be made to the Court of Protection for a statutory will. Whether this is done is a matter for the person's solicitor, bearing in mind the cost of such an application.

As above, as only a testator can write a will, this cannot be deferred to a healthcare professional (C).

In this situation the capacity relates to a will and therefore testamentary capacity should be assessed (D). Mental capacity relates to the Mental Capacity Act 2005 which came into force in 2007, sets out the clear legal requirements for assessing capacity in adults aged over 18 years old, and may also be used in those aged 16–17 whose incompetence is likely to persist into adulthood. A person lacks capacity if they fail any one of the following criteria: (1) understanding the information relevant to the decision; (2) retaining the information (even if only for a short period); (3) using or weighing that information; or (4) communicating the decision (by any means).

→ Jacoby R (2007). How to assess capacity to make a will. *British Medical Journal*, **335**, 155–7.

2. B ★   OHPsych 3rd edn → pp.882–3

To be discharged from sections 2 and 3 of the MHA, the patient has to be discharged by the Responsible Clinician (RC), a Mental Health Tribunal, or hospital managers (B).

GPs may be involved in sectioning patients, usually as one of the supporting medical recommendations. However, they do not have the power to discharge patients from section (A).

The medical director does not have the authority to discharge the patient from section (C).

The NR can make an application for discharge from section. However, this can be barred by the RC (D).

Any ward doctor would not be allowed to discharge the patient from section (E), although the RC would be allowed to.

3. A ★   OHPsych 3rd edn → pp.874–5

The correct answer is to give antipsychotic medication under the MHA (A). The MHA allows for treatment of mental disorder without the patient's consent. In this case it would be important to treat her mental disorder in the first instance and ensure that her mental state is stabilized. Once mental state is stabilized it would be important to assess her reason for not accepting treatment for HIV and determine whether or not she has capacity to refuse treatment. Under the terms of the Mental Capacity Act 2005, all adults are presumed to have sufficient capacity to decide on their own medical treatment unless there is significant evidence to suggest otherwise. If she does have capacity, treatment cannot be given against her will, even if it is felt that she is making an unwise decision. If she does not have capacity, the doctor should check to see if there is an attorney or other legal proxy appointed to make healthcare decisions for the patient. The doctor must also involve members of the healthcare team and those close to the patient. If contested, the Courts may have to decide on treatment.

Covert medication can sometimes be given under the MHA for the treatment of mental disorder but not physical disorder (B).

Medication for physical health problems cannot be given under the MHA unless the physical disorder arises from the mental disorder (C).

Whilst antipsychotic medication can sometimes be given covertly under the MHA (usually with the approval of a second-opinion doctor), antiretrovirals could not be given in this way (D).

Although antipsychotics could be given under the MHA, antiretrovirals could not be given under the MHA as HIV is a physical disorder (and has not arisen from the mental disorder) (E).

→ Jones R (2012). *Mental Health Act Manual*, 15th edn. Sweet and Maxwell, London.

4. E ★   OHPsych 3rd edn → pp.902–3

If the patient has a condition or is on medication that makes driving unsafe and the patient is unable to appreciate this, or refuses to cease driving, the GMC recommends breaking confidentiality and informing the DVLA. The guidelines state that before contacting the DVLA doctors should inform the patient of their decision to disclose personal information, and should also inform the patient in writing once they have made the disclosure (E).

It is correct to inform the DVLA in this situation. However, GMC guidelines state you should try to inform the patient that you are going to disclose information to the DVLA (A). This does not mean that the patient can stop you, just that they are aware of what you are doing.

Telling the patient's employer (B) breaches patient confidentiality and is not in line with GMC recommendations, which state that the DVLA should be informed.

As the patient continues to drive when they may not be fit to do so, the doctors have a professional duty to inform the DVLA. Patients should be aware that their driving licence is invalid whilst on a methadone treatment programme unless agreed by the DVLA following receipt of supportive medical advice. So for this patient to drive would be illegal. It would be appropriate to inform the police (C) if the patient was felt to be unfit to drive following the consumption of methadone, but this is supplemental to informing the DVLA.

Stopping the methadone (D) might result in the patient using heroin to relieve cravings, which would be more harmful to the patient and potentially the public if he continued to work.

→ GMC Supplementary Guidance—Confidentiality: reporting concerns about patients to the DVLA or the DVA, September 2009: http://www.gmc-uk.org/Confidentiality_reporting_concerns_DVLA_2009.pdf?dm_i=OUY,1JCHI,3F9130,595N3,1.

5. E ★★ OHPsych 3rd edn → pp.898–901

There are certain situations where a doctor should break the normal confidentiality agreement between doctor and patient. One of these is to assist in the prevention of a serious crime, where someone may be at risk of death or serious injury—see Tarasoff case (OHPsych 3rd edn → p.901. In this case the patient cannot be relied on to inform the police. The threat he has made is of serious harm to another person and therefore steps should be made to warn third parties of threatened danger arising from a patient's violent intentions. In the absence of having no contact information for the potential victim the most appropriate course of action is to inform the police (E).

Whilst he should be aware of what you plan, breaking confidentiality and informing the police does not require his permission (A). In this case, it would be fair to tell him that there will be a conversation with the police but not to ask his 'permission' for this to take place.

This should be documented as first-person information as he has stated it directly to the doctor. Information that is related to the patient and supplied by another person, professional, or agency or has been treated as confidential by the said third party, can be said to be third party information (B).

Despite the fact that he has requested that this information is not recorded, he has made a threat of serious harm to someone and this cannot be ignored. The patient should be informed that this information has to be recorded in his notes and due to the nature of the disclosure it is not possible to keep the information confidential (C).

It is not appropriate, or relevant, to inform the NR (D). There is a duty of care to the ex-girlfriend (and anyone else in danger), but it is not the patient's relative's responsibility to challenge this.

6. C ★★   OHPsych 3rd edn → pp.874–5

Dealing with the acute situation will require rapid tranquillization (C), and following this an assessment under the MHA would be appropriate as the patient is posing as a harm to others, suffering from a mental disorder, and not consenting to treatment.

The patient is being physically aggressive in response to delusional beliefs. The situation may escalate further, so watchful waiting is likely to be hazardous in this situation (A).

In this scenario the priority is safe, effective treatment rather than organizing MHA assessments. This would be the next appropriate step once the situation is safer and more settled (B).

Decisions made in good faith by medical staff in the acute situation, taken to avert serious risk, can be sanctioned by common law without recourse to the Mental Capacity Act (D).

As the patient is not detained, a section 62 for emergency powers of treatment is not applicable (E).

→ Mental Capacity Act 2005 Code of Practice (2007 Final Edition): http://www.justice.gov.uk/protecting-the-vulnerable/mental-capacity-act. .

7. C ★★   OHPsych 3rd edn → pp.880–3

The most appropriate is Section 4 (emergency admission) (C). This allows a patient to be admitted in an emergency only in patients who have not yet been admitted to hospital (it includes those in the ED, outpatient clinic, and day hospitals). It lasts up to 72 hours and must be signed by a doctor and an approved mental health professional. It is not commonly used. It is appropriate in this scenario because of the acute presentation of the man coupled with the risk he poses, together with the likely delay in finding a second doctor to complete the other medical recommendation for admission. Section 4 orders can be 'converted' to a section 2 when in hospital, based on another recommendation for formal admission from a second doctor. As this is just used for assessment, the patient cannot be treated against their will with this order.

Section 2 (admission for assessment) (A) requires an application for detention made by the NR or the approved mental health professional and requires two medical recommendations, one of which must be an approved doctor.

Application for a section 3 (admission for treatment) (B) is made in a similar manner to section 2.

Section 5(2) (D) is the doctor's holding power. The doctor in charge of the patient's care (or a nominated deputy, which is often the duty doctor) states how the criteria for detention are met and reasons why informal treatment is no longer appropriate. Section 5(2) can be used in both a psychiatric hospital and a general hospital and lasts up to 72 hours.

Section 5(4) (E) is the nurse's holding power. It allows a suitably qualified nurse to detain an informal patient in hospital for up to six hours for a medical assessment. In order to be used it must not be practicable to get a doctor to attend who might place the patient on section 5(2). Section 5(4) is not renewable. The holding power ends as soon as a doctor arrives.

8. C ★★   OHPsych 3rd edn → pp.870–3

A patient detained in hospital (except under emergency provisions) may be given medication for mental disorder for up to three months, whether they consent or not and/or have the capacity. It is appropriate to treat his psychosis despite his refusal to take oral medication (C).

It is not appropriate to give patients medications covertly (A). If this patient requires treatment that he is not agreeing to take orally, he should be given it in IM form.

As this patient was recently detained it is not necessary to get a second opinion regarding antipsychotic medication (B). Under section 58, medication for over three months requires the patient's consent or, if the patient refuses or is incapable, agreement of a second-opinion approved doctor.

Under section 62, treatment that is urgently necessary may be authorized by the RC without consent or a second opinion, whilst awaiting a second opinion (D).

This patient is detained in hospital and acutely unwell. He requires treatment, and waiting for him to agree to take oral medications is not in his best interests (E). Treating his psychotic symptoms is of paramount importance.

9. A ★★★★   OHPsych 3rd edn → p.887

The most appropriate treatment is to add lithium as an adjunct to her antidepressant medication (A). The Mental Capacity Act makes it possible for someone who is over 18 years old and has mental capacity to do this to make an advance decision to refuse specified treatment should they lack capacity in the future. Advance decisions cannot demand specific treatments, but they can refuse treatment and state the person's wishes regarding treatment options. Changes to the MHA in 2007 mean that it is no longer possible to give ECT against the patient's will if they are capable of consenting. It may still be given if the patient is unable to consent, provided there is no prior advance decision. In this scenario, optimal medical management has not been tried yet, so that would be the appropriate next step.

If there is a valid advance decision against ECT, this cannot be overridden by doctors except in an emergency (B). If the patient were to stop eating/drinking, for example, then it might be appropriate in that situation to give emergency ECT.

As above, as there is a valid advance decision against ECT, this cannot be overridden by doctors except in an emergency (C).

Advance decisions may not be applicable if the advance decision refuses treatment for a mental disorder and the person is detained under the MHA (D). The exception to this is with ECT. However, ECT may be given appropriately, against the advance decision, if it were an emergency.

A relative cannot give permission for ECT to be given to this patient (E).

→ Mental Capacity Act 2005 Code of Practice (2007 Final Edition) http://www.justice.gov.uk/protecting-the-vulnerable/mental-capacity-act.

10. A ★★★★   OHPsych 3rd edn → pp.880–1

The NR has a number or powers and responsibilities, including the right to: (1) apply for detention or guardianship; (2) object to approved mental health professionals making applications for admission to hospital; (3) ask that their relative be assessed under the MHA and receive written information if the decision is taken not to admit that person; (4) discharge patients or to apply to the Mental Health Review Tribunal. The NR can be displaced by application to the Court, which can be made by the patient, any relative of the patient (see list below), anyone who lives with the patient, or an approved mental health professional (A).

Hospital managers are not allowed to apply for displacement of the NR (B).

Detaining the person against the wishes of the NR would not be lawful (C). An application to the Court would need to be made for the NR to be displaced.

If this patient were not detained and instead treated in the community (D), it would not be safe for the patient or other people. In this case there is grounds to displace the NR as they are seemingly objecting unreasonably to admission. Other grounds for displacement of the NR include: there is no NR, the NR is too ill to take on the role, or the NR has discharged the patient without regard to that person's (or other people's) safety.

The NR is usually determined by who is first on the following list: husband, wife, or civil partner (includes people living with a patient as a couple for at least six months prior to hospital admission), son or daughter, father or mother, brother or sister, grandparent, grandchild, uncle or aunt, nephew or niece, a person who has ordinarily been residing with the patient for five years or more. Within each category, male and female relatives are treated equally, with the older person being given priority (E).

Extended Matching Questions

1. J ★★

Section 136 relates to the powers allowing the police to take a mentally disordered person to a place of safety.

2. C ★★

Section 5(2) relates to the emergency detention of a hospital inpatient by a doctor (usually the duty doctor), lasting up to 72 hours. Involvement of a social worker or NR is not necessary.

3. G ★★

Section 47 relates to the transfer of a sentenced prisoner (rather than a pre-sentence prisoner which would be a section 48) from prison to hospital.

4. F ★★

Section 37 relates to a mental health disposal following conviction. A hospital order (rather than a section 3, for example) is given to a mentally disordered offender at time of sentencing.

5. A ★★

This question relates to the application of a section for further assessment. The patient is not known to services and has no previous psychiatric history; therefore a section 2 is more appropriate than a section 3 in this case.

General feedback on 1–5: OHPsych 3rd edn → pp.880–3

6. H ★★★★

There were exclusions in the MHA 1983 that a person should not be treated as suffering from mental disorder by reason only of:

- Promiscuity or other immoral conduct
- Sexual deviancy
- Dependence on alcohol or drugs.

This was amended in the MHA 2007 to:

- His substance misuse (including dependence on alcohol or drugs)
- His sexual identity or orientation
- His commission or likely commission of illegal or disorderly acts
- His cultural, religious, or political beliefs.

Dependence on alcohol or drugs is therefore not considered to be a disorder or disability of mind. This exclusion refers to dependence only; therefore other mental disorders relating to the use of alcohol or drugs are not excluded, e.g. withdrawal state with delirium or associated psychotic disorder or even severe acute intoxication, provided all the relevant criteria for detention under the MHA are met.

7. G ★★★★

People with learning disabilities are ineligible for detention under long-term powers of detention unless their learning disability is associated with abnormally aggressive or seriously irresponsible conduct.

8. G ★★★★

As for Item 1, a person should not be treated as suffering from mental disorder by reason only of sexual deviancy; however, some disorders of sexual preference are recognized clinically as mental disorders, such as paraphilias, fetishism, or paedophilia, and are included in the ICD-10. Under the 1983 MHA a person could only be detained if suffering from mental illness, psychopathic disorder, mental impairment, or severe mental impairment. The MHA 2007 abolished the four separate categories of mental disorder and stated that a person could be detained if suffering from any disorder or disability of mind, meaning that patients suffering from a disorder of sexual preference could be detained under the Act.

9. B ★★★★

People who lack the capacity to consent now benefit from safeguards covering both care homes and those being treated in hospital, in circumstances where their need to receive care or treatment amounts to a deprivation of liberty. In past situations, such as some people with severe dementia or autism, these people have been 'detained' under the common law, rather than under the MHA, and so did not have sufficient legal safeguards or protection. Changes were made in response to the 2004 European Court of Human Rights' judgement involving an autistic man who was kept at Bournewood Hospital by doctors against the wishes of his carers. The Court found that he had been deprived of his liberty unlawfully and there was a lack of procedural safeguards regulating the admission. The Department of Health committed to introducing new legislation to close what has come to be known as the 'Bournewood gap'. The Deprivation of Liberty Safeguards are the attempt by the Government to bridge the Bournewood gap, so that all those lacking capacity deprived of their liberty have safeguards consistent with the requirements of Article 5 of the Human Rights Act.

10. G ★★★★

Under the MHA 1983 a person with a PD could only be detained if it fulfilled the criteria for the legal category of psychopathic disorder, meaning a persistent disorder or disability of mind that results in abnormally aggressive or seriously irresponsible conduct. The broader definition of mental disorder under the MHA 2007 (any disorder or disability of mind) allows for all PDs to be included and removes the requirement of abnormally aggressive or seriously irresponsible requirement in cases of PD.

General feedback on 6–10: OHPsych 3rd edn → pp.870–7

→ Mental Health Act 1983: revised Code of Practice: http://www.legislation.gov.uk/ukpga/2007/12/contents.

Chapter 9

Child and adolescent psychiatry

Louise Morganstein and Jonathan Hill

Child and adolescent psychiatry is the medical specialty that works with children, young people, and families with emotional and behavioural problems. As children and young people are still developing and growing, their emotional wellbeing and functioning needs to be thought about in this context, making it different from adult psychiatry.

Communication with people of all ages is vital within the specialty and information from a wide variety of sources, including parents or carers, school, and peers, is used to inform the clinical picture, in addition to history-taking and direct observations of the child's behaviour. Play is often used to understand younger children's thoughts and feelings. In theory, the specialty covers children and young people from birth up to the teenage years, although different services cover slightly different age ranges.

The spectrum of difficulties covered within the specialty include psychiatric disorders also seen in adults (such as psychosis); problems specific to the age group (such as separation anxiety); lifelong conditions which start in childhood (such as ADHD); and conditions that may present in different ways in childhood or adolescence (such as phobias).

Approaches to treatment include psychopharmacological interventions, and numerous therapeutic modalities including family therapy and CBT, which can be modified for different age groups. Most work is community based, although there are specialist inpatient units which offer on-going educational opportunities to young people who need the intensive support and risk reduction of a hospital admission. Work tends to be done within MDTs using a range of knowledge and expertise to offer the most appropriate care.

Louise Morganstein

QUESTIONS

Single Best Answers

1. A 15-year-old adolescent has had low mood, loss of interest in her usual activities, and no hope for the future for the past month. Which *single* somatic symptom is she most likely to report? ★

A Abdominal pain

B Headache

C Increased thirst

D Loss of appetite

E Shortness of breath

2. A four-year-old child has delayed speech. He has a particular interest in trains and enjoys lining them up in straight lines. He does not look the doctor in the eye for more than a few seconds. Which is the *single* most likely diagnosis? ★

A ADHD

B ASD

C Dyspraxia

D Fragile X

E Specific language delay

3. An 11-year-old girl is having trouble sleeping. She is due to start secondary school in a few weeks. Her mother takes her to the GP for advice. General reassurance has already been given. Which is the *single* most appropriate management? ★

A Family therapy

B PRN sedative antihistamine

C Review in two weeks

D Sleep hygiene advice

E Sleeping tablets for one week

4. A nine-year-old child with moderate ADHD continues to fidget a lot in lessons and shouts out answers. His teachers feel that his condition is interfering with his education. His parents have attended a structured parenting course. Which is the *single* most appropriate next management step? ★

A Atomoxetine

B CBT

C Family sessions

D Methylphenidate

E No additional treatment

5. A 14-year-old adolescent has OCD. She repeatedly counts her belongings and checks whether she has turned light switches off. She is keen to have the best evidence-based treatment available. Which is the *single* most appropriate treatment? ★

A Antipsychotic medication

B Benzodiazepine medication

C Cognitive analytical therapy

D Exposure and response prevention treatment

E Individual psychodynamic psychotherapy

6. A 16-year-old adolescent is in the ED after taking a paracetamol overdose. Her named nurse asks what she should ask about to help predict any future risk of further episodes of self-harm. Which is the *single* most appropriate answer to give? ★

A Whether her friends have ever overdosed

B Whether she has a history of previous DSH

C Whether she took the tablets with alcohol

D Whether she tried to conceal taking this overdose

E Whether she wrote a suicide note

7. A 15-year-old adolescent has been referred to his school counsellor who is concerned he may be depressed. The counsellor has asked about his symptoms. Which is the *single* most relevant piece of additional information to ask? ★

A Academic history

B Family medical history

C Parental mental health problems

D Predicted exam grades

E Religious beliefs

8. A ten-year-old boy is still wetting the bed at night on a regular basis. He is upset about this behaviour as it is preventing him from staying over at friends' houses. Which is the *single* most appropriate management? ★★

A Alarmed mattress

B A reward system

C Fluid restriction after 6 pm

D Lifting onto the toilet during sleep

E Vasopressin

9. The mother of a ten-year-old child has been reading about emotional problems and mental health difficulties among children and young people. She has read they are 'common' between the ages of one and fifteen but is unsure what this means. Which is the *single* most accurate way of describing this prevalence? ★★

A 1 in 5 children

B 1 in 10 children

C 1 in 20 children

D 1 in 50 children

E 1 in 100 children

10. A 16-year-old adolescent with anorexia nervosa is referred for treatment. She has two sisters both of whom are younger and are being affected by her difficulties. Which is the *single* most appropriate initial management? ★★★

A Family therapy

B IPT

C Paediatric assessment of siblings

D Social services referral

E SSRI prescription

11. A seven-year-old girl had a tooth removed a month ago. The procedure was painful and she found it very distressing. Since then she has been worried about opening her mouth and has slowly stopped eating and drinking. In the last two days she has only had sips of water. Which is the *single* most appropriate next step? ★★★

A Calculate her BMI

B CBT

C Check her BP

D Family therapy

E U&Es

12. A three-year-old child started going to nursery six months ago. He refuses to go and still cries for three hours when he is dropped off by his mother. Over the weekend he frequently asks his parents where they are going when they leave the room and seems worried that they won't come back. He struggles to get to sleep unless his mother lies down next to him and holds his hand, and cries if this routine doesn't happen. His parents are very concerned by his behaviour and say that it is stopping them from doing everyday things like going out for a meal as a couple. Which is the *single* most likely diagnosis? ★★★

A Adjustment disorder

B Generalized anxiety disorder

C Normal behaviour

D Separation anxiety disorder

E Social phobia

13. A five-year-old boy frequently gets frightened and asks his mother if he will be "OK". She is concerned that this is something she has done wrong or that she has unwittingly exposed him to a scary situation. Which is the *single* most likely normal fear in a child this age? ★★★

A Being around other people

B Clowns

C Crowds

D Spiders

E The dark

14. A 15-year-old adolescent is referred to the MDT. He has a history of sexual abuse and emotional difficulties. After a full assessment it is agreed that his management plan should include some form of long-term talking treatment. Which *single* professional is the most appropriate to offer this treatment? ★★★★

A Child and adolescent psychotherapist

B Counselling psychologist

C Registered mental health nurse

D Children's social worker

E Speech and language therapist

Extended Matching Questions

Diagnosis of child and adolescent psychiatric problems

For each of the following patients, choose the *single* most likely diagnosis from the list of options below. Each option may be used once, more than once, or not at all. ★

A ADHD

B Asperger's syndrome

C Bulimia nervosa

D Conduct disorder

E Emotionally unstable PD

F Encopresis

G Enuresis

H Generalized learning disability

I Oppositional defiant disorder

J Simple tic disorder

1. A 14-year-old adolescent repeatedly has episodes where she eats multiple bags of crisps, biscuits, and bread before feeling sick and forcing herself to vomit. Her BMI is 24 kg/m^2.

2. A 15-year-old adolescent has been in trouble with the police on a few occasions and frequently gets in trouble at school for bullying others. He does not seem to listen to his teachers or parents and was in a fight last night.

3. A 12-year-old boy frequently moves his head to the left without noticing that he is doing it. When it is pointed out to him he can stop doing it for a short time but cannot stop for prolonged periods. His neck examination is normal.

4. A six-year-old girl has just started a new school and has begun to soil herself during the day. Before this she was out of nappies and dry in the daytime and at night. She has not had any gastrointestinal infections.

5. A nine-year-old boy is struggling to keep up at school. He has always found learning difficult and is behind in all of his classes. He has recently seen an educational psychologist for an assessment.

Mangement of child and adolescent psychiatric problems

For each of the following patients, choose the *single* most appropriate management. Each option may be used once, more than once, or not at all.★★

A Anger management

B Antipsychotic medication

C Body image focused therapy

D CBT

E Family group conference

F IPT

G Parenting skills training programme

H Positive behavioural reinforcement and rewards using star charts

I SSRI prescription

J Structured calorie-counted meal plan

6. An 11-year-old boy who is often stubborn and angry has been suspended from school following numerous detentions over recent months for breaking the rules. His teachers report that he blames other pupils when he gets in trouble and argues back when he is told off. He is easily annoyed and is struggling to make friends.

7. A 17-year-old adolescent with a diagnosis of moderately severe depression has completed a course of CBT. She returns to see you in clinic saying that she still feels low in mood and wants to know what else you can offer.

8. A 16-year-old adolescent presents with paranoid thoughts that his peers are trying to poison him. On further questioning he seems to really believe that this is happening to him and can't be persuaded that there is another explanation. He is worried about going to school because of this.

9. A 14-year-old adolescent has been losing weight for the past few months. She is struggling to know what she should be eating, as she thinks she is overweight and wants to be slimmer. Her mother reports that she has been throwing her packed lunch away at school. She hasn't had a period for the past two months. Her blood results are normal.

10. An eight-year-old boy with a mild learning disability has been getting in trouble for throwing food at home during mealtimes. His parents want help to change his behaviour.

ANSWERS

Single Best Answers

1. D ★
OHPsych 3rd edn → p.652

Although all of these symptoms can be associated with depression and anxiety, loss of appetite (D) is the most commonly associated with low mood. It is important to ask about weight change in addition to appetite change and this may require some further investigation.

Abdominal pain (A) and headache (B) are often reported by young people experiencing anxiety and frequently used as a reason not to go to school. Either may be a feature of depression but this is less common.

Increased thirst (C) can be a symptom of diabetes mellitus, and if associated with other symptoms should be investigated. It is not a common somatic symptom of depression but can be a side-effect of medication.

Shortness of breath (E) may be a sign of panic or anxiety. It should always be taken seriously, as underlying causes like asthma may need to be ruled out.

→ YoungMinds: What is depression? http://www.youngminds.org.uk/for_children_young_people/whats_worrying_you/depression/what_is_depression.

2. B ★
OHPsych 3rd edn → pp.630–1

The most likely diagnosis is ASD (B). The three main features of autism are language delay, restricted and repetitive interests, and social communication difficulties.

The main features of ADHD (A) are hyperactivity, inattention, and impulsivity.

Dyspraxia (C) is also known as developmental coordination disorder. It affects movement and coordination but not social communication. It is thought to be due to an uncoordinated response to a common stimulus between left and right hemispheres of the brain.

Fragile X (D) is a genetic condition characterized by intellectual impairment, a long face and large ears, flat feet, hyperextensible joints, and frequently emotional and behavioural problems.

For a diagnosis of specific language delay (E) there should not be any additional symptoms such as lack of eye contact or restricted interest. Specific language impairment is a language difficulty that interferes with daily life or academic progress and performance on a standardized language test which is significantly below the child's age level. All other causes should have been excluded, for example the problems cannot be explained in terms of hearing loss or a physical difficulty.

→ Autistic spectrum disorder: http://www.nhs.uk/conditions/autistic-spectrum-disorder/Pages/Introduction.aspx.

→ Map of medicine—autism in children: http://healthguides.mapof-medicine.com/choices/map/autism_spectrum_disorder_asd_in_children1.html.

→ National Autistic Society—diagnosing autism: http://www.autism.org.uk/About-autism/All-about-diagnosis/Diagnosis-the-process-for-children.aspx.

3. C ★   OHPsych 3rd edn → pp.638, 665

The answer is review in two weeks (C). In the short term general reassurance is all that is needed. Changes in routine can be anxiety provoking, particularly for young people who may have limited experience of change. Worries can result in physical symptoms in children and young people, such as disturbed sleep, abdominal pain, and headaches.

This is a normal reaction to change and family therapy is not indicated at this time (A). It is important to ensure that common difficulties are not pathologized and that the young person does not take on an illness role.

Medication (B) is rarely prescribed for sleep problems in young people. Not only would the side-effect profile need to be taken into account, but also, in general, it is felt that young people learning to manage their symptoms without medical support leads to better long-term outcome measures.

If the problem persists then sleep hygiene advice may be appropriate (D), but not in the first instance. Within the NHS it is important that consideration is taken to offer a pragmatic treatment plan which takes into account that normal reactions are not medicalized or labelled as a disorder.

Medication is rarely prescribed for sleep problems in young people. In this instance, a week-long prescription (E) may mask the problem or even exacerbate it with rebound symptoms activation.

→ NHS—Sleep hygiene advice: http://www.nhs.uk/Conditions/Insomnia/Pages/Prevention.aspx.

4. D ★   OHPsych 3rd edn → pp.628–9

Methylphenidate (D) is the first-line medication. It would initially be prescribed as short-acting doses to get the dose right and could then be converted into longer-acting preparations.

As his parents have already been on a structured parenting course the next step is to offer medication, of which the first line is methylphenidate not atomoxetine (A).

CBT (B) is not recommended in the treatment of ADHD.

Family sessions (C) are not indicated in this scenario—medication is the next step.

This young boy's ADHD is getting in the way of his education, and therefore doing nothing isn't an option (E).

→ NICE Clinical Guideline 72—ADHD: http://www.nice.org.uk/CG72.

5. D ★   OHPsych 3rd edn → pp.648–9

OCD can be treated with both psychological therapy and SSRI medication. The first-line treatment is CBT, of which one type is known as exposure and response prevention treatment (D). In this, patients are exposed to the things that make them anxious (obsessions) and learn to cope with the anxiety without using their compulsive behaviours to reduce the anxiety.

Antipsychotic medication (A) is not indicated in the first line-treatment of OCD. It is more commonly used to treat psychosis.

Benzodiazepines (B) are rarely used in children and adolescents aside from the acute treatment of mania and agitation. They are not useful in the longer-term management of OCD.

CAT (C) is not a first-line recommended treatment for OCD. It is a time-limited therapy focusing on repeating maladaptive patterns. It includes the therapist writing a letter to the patient.

Individual psychodynamic therapy (E) is usually used as a long-term therapy, looking into the past to understand why and how individuals function in the present. It is not a first-line treatment for OCD.

→ NICE Clinical Guideline 31—OCD: http://publications.nice.org.uk/obsessive-compulsive-disorder-cg31/guidance,stepped-care-for-adults-young-people-and-children-with-ocd-or-bdd.

6. B ★   OHPsych 3rd edn → pp.654–5

Although all of the options are useful questions and may inform your clinical view of the severity of the current situation, the single biggest predictor of future risk is a past history of self-harm (B).

Knowledge of her friendship group is important; however, this is not generally a predictor of future risk (A). Occasionally there are pacts around self-harm or suicide which are important to recognize, but the reality of 'suicide pacts' is that they are covered in the media (both fact and fiction) more than they occur in real life. There is evidence to suggest that some youth subcultures, such as 'goths', normalize DSH, making it more likely that someone will experiment with these actions without any mental illness.

Understanding the circumstances of the current overdose allows one to understand the intention behind it and the seriousness of the intent, but this is not the best predictor of future risk. Taking an overdose with alcohol (C) can impact on the management of the overdose and also how the initial history is taken, as the patient may still be drunk or hung over, as well as emotional about the overdose itself.

Concealing an overdose (D) is dangerous in itself as it may prevent, or at least slow, treatment. However, the most useful predictor of future events is past patterns. In some cases there may have been undisclosed overdoses, sometimes minor enough to be written off as 'accidental' or simply ignored by the patient, which have never been reported. This is different from active concealment but would nonetheless better fit into a pattern of previous DSH.

Writing a suicide note (E) is serious but will not necessarily help to predict future events. As mentioned, understanding the current overdose situation highlights the current intentions but can be biased toward current stressors. In this context, it is worth considering the 'suicide note' in the context of that person's life, as a handwritten note may be very different from a short, angry SMS (short message service) or a status update about suicide which garners lots of attention.

→ NICE Clinical Guideline 16—Self-harm: http://publications.nice.org. uk/self-harm-cg16/guidance.

7. C ★   OHPsych 3rd edn → pp.652–3

According to NICE guidance on depression in children and young people, 'consideration should be given to the possibility of parental depression, parental substance misuse, or other mental health problems...as these are often associated with depression in a child or young person and, if untreated, may have a negative impact on the success of treatment offered to the child or young person' (C).

Information about academic history (A), and all social circumstances, is part of a proper history. It may be necessary to liaise with current and past schools in the future, but this information is unlikely to impact an initial formulation.

It is important to know about a family medical history (B) when it comes to prescribing medication, especially a family history of high BP, but it not be important in diagnosis or making an initial formulation.

Exam stress can impact on young people's mood and behaviour (D). Knowing specific information like this is unlikely to impact an initial formulation. However, it could be included in a formulation about the predisposing, precipitating, and prolonging factors behind the depression.

Religious beliefs (E) can impact on young people's thoughts. It is helpful to consider this when planning management, but knowing specific information like this is unlikely to impact an initial formulation.

→ NICE Clinical Guideline 28— Depression in Children and Young People: http://publications.nice.org.uk/depression-in-children-and-yo ung-people-cg28/guidance.

8. B ★★   OHPsych 3rd edn → p.636

A reward system for an agreed behaviour should be the first treatment offered (B). This allows the child to gain control of the situation and helps them learn to change their behaviour.

Secondary treatments include the use of alarmed mattresses (A). This is seen as using punishment (i.e. waking the child up) which is effective but not preferred.

Fluid restriction (C) is not advised, although excessive intake can be addressed. Ensuring an adequate but not excessive daily fluid intake must take into account ambient temperature, dietary intake, and physical activity.

Lifting children to go to the toilet (D) only offers short-term management and not a long-term solution.

Medication in children is avoided as a first-line treatment (E). Behavioural techniques are favoured as they offer long-term solutions and avoid medication side-effects.

→ NICE Clinical Guideline 111—Nocturnal enuresis: http://publications.nice.org.uk/nocturnal-enuresis-cg111.

9. B ★★   OHPsych 3rd edn → pp.610, 639

One in ten children between the ages of one and fifteen has a mental health disorder (B).

The figure of 1 in 5 children (A) is too high for prevalence, although research suggests that 20% of children have a mental health problem in any given year.

Answers (C), (D), and (E) are all too low—mental health problems in children and young people are more common than this.

→ Green H, McGinnity A, Meltzer H, Ford T, Goodman R (2005). *Mental Health of Children and Young People in Great Britain, 2004*. Palgrave Macmillan, Basingstoke.

→ Mental Health Foundation—Mental Health Statistics: Children & Young People: http://www.mentalhealth.org.uk/help-information/mental-health-statistics/children-young-people/.

10. A ★★★   OHPsych 3rd edn → p.666

Family therapy (A) has a strong evidence base in the treatment of anorexia nervosa. Siblings should be included in family therapy, as the impact on their lives can be significant.

IPT (B) focuses on relationships with others and on communication difficulties. NICE recommends IPT for individuals with eating disorders, but the siblings are not usually seen.

Based on the information available, there is no need to assess the siblings in their own right (C), but involving them in family therapy may be helpful.

Based on the information available, there is no need to involve social services (D), although if there are concerns that the siblings' needs are not being met this may become a child protection case.

SSRIs (E) may be used in treating co-morbid depression.

→ B-eat (Beating Eating Disorders): http://www.b-eat-carers.co.uk/siblings/.

→ NICE Clinical Guideline 9—Eating disorders: http://guidance.nice.org.uk/CG9.

11. E ★★★   OHPsych 3rd edn → p.644

Blood tests to measure dehydration and electrolyte imbalance are the most urgent as life-saving treatment may be needed (E).

BMI (A) only gives a calculation of weight and height. It does not include information about hydration.

Although addressing this child's emotional response to a painful procedure will be intrinsic to longer-term treatment, it is vital that any dehydration is recognized and treated immediately, as this could be fatal if left unrecognized. CBT (B) or family therapy (D) could be considered once the child is well and in a physically safe condition—the type of therapy would depend on the patient and the family's needs at that time.

The most immediately concerning consequence in this scenario is dehydration. Although a BP measurement (C) can give an indication of current hydration level it is not as useful as blood tests in measuring the degree of dehydration and/or electrolyte imbalance. In practice, baseline observations, including BP, should be done routinely.

→ NHS—Dehydration in Children: Map of Medicine: http://health-guides.mapofmedicine.com/choices/map/dehydration_in_children1.html.

12. D ★★★   OHPsych 3rd edn → pp.620–1

This is a typical separation anxiety disorder (D). It is important to be clear of the difference between the disorder and separation anxiety which is normal in children aged around one year of age.

This is not an adjustment disorder (A) as there is no significant stressor aside from starting nursery, which most children cope well with given time.

This is not a generalized anxiety disorder (B) as the anxiety is focused around separating from his parents.

This presentation could be normal behaviour (C) in the first few weeks of starting nursery, but should resolve itself as the child becomes more used to their new environment and learns that their parents consistently collect them each day.

This is not social phobia (E) as the anxiety is focused around separating from his parents and not being around other people or performing. Social phobia is unusual in such a young child.

→ Boston Children's Hospital—Separation Anxiety Disorder: http://www.childrenshospital.org/az/Site1573/mainpageS1573P1.html.

→ RCPsych information on anxiety in young people: http://www.rcpsych.ac.uk/expertadvice/youthinfo/parentscarers/growingup/worriesandanxieties.aspx.

13. E ★★★   OHPsych 3rd edn → pp.644–5

Being afraid of the dark (E) is a common fear for young children. It should not initially be thought about as a phobia unless it is persistent or the child cannot be reassured.

It is normal for children to have certain fears as they grow up. These are not phobias and usually disappear with reassurance and time. Social phobia, or the fear of being around others (A) or social interactions, can occur in young people but is more common in adolescence.

There is a specific phobia of clowns (B), coulrophobia, but this is unlikely in a child of this age. However, the noise and unexpected movements of clowns can sometimes be frightening to children.

There is a specific phobia of crowds (C) and open spaces, agoraphobia, but this is unlikely in a child of this age.

There is a specific phobia of spiders (D), arachnophobia, but this is unlikely in a child of this age.

→ Healthvisitors.com—The Stages of Emotional Development From 0–5 Years: http://www.healthvisitors.com/parents/stages_emotional_development.htm.

→ Zero to Three—Toddlers' fears: http://www.zerotothree.org/child-development/social-emotional-development/qa/my-2-year-old-son-is-suddenly.html

14. A ★★★★   OHPsych 3rd edn → p.621

A typical CAMHS team will have a number of different disciplines represented, including psychiatry, psychology, nursing, and professionals trained in various psychotherapies. Child and adolescent psychotherapists (A) have specialist skills in working with young people with complex emotional and behavioural needs, and those exposed to abuse.

Counselling psychologists (B) generally work with adults, not young people. According to NHS Choices, the role of a counselling psychologist is to 'work collaboratively with people, to treat a wide range of issues, including helping people manage difficult life events (such as bereavement), past and present relationships and helping people with mental health issues and disorders'.

Registered mental health nurses (C) can be part of CAMHS teams, but unless they have additional training they are unlikely to undertake complex or longer-term therapy.

This also applies to social workers (D).

Speech and language therapists (E) often work closely with CAMHS teams, but would not be indicated in this case.

→ RCPsych information on who's who in CAMHS: http://www.rcpsych.ac.uk/healthadvice/parentsandyouthinfo/parentscarers/whoswhoincamhs.aspx

→ Young Minds—Who works in CAMHS? http://www.youngminds.org.uk/for_parents/services_children_young_people/camhs/who_works_in_camhs.

Extended Matching Questions

1. C ★

Bulimia nervosa is an eating disorder characterized by frequent binges and then purges. Sufferers are usually normal weight. Anorexia is not the correct answer as sufferers are low weight.

2. D ★

Conduct disorder is a condition characterized by repeated antisocial behaviours. This is the most appropriate answer in this case, although in an assessment other conditions such as ADHD and Asperger's syndrome (high functioning ASD) would need to be thought about as these may contribute to conduct disordered behaviour. Oppositional defiant disorder presents in a similar way to conduct disorder but is with younger children and less serious behaviours.

3. J ★

A simple tic involves the involuntary movement of a single muscle group. None of the other answers involves problematic single movements. ADHD presents with overactivity but this is not isolated to a single movement. ASD (including Asperger's syndrome) can present with unusual movements, such as flapping arms, but you would need other symptoms, such as social communication difficulties, before making a diagnosis.

4. F ★

Encopresis is faecal soiling. It can either start after successful toilet training or be diagnosed when no toilet training has been achieved by an age when it should have been. Although it is easy to confuse the two conditions, enuresis refers to urinary incontinence only. Other conditions such as generalized learning difficulty can be associated with toileting problems, but there are more likely to be difficulties gaining continence in the first place.

5. H ★

The most likely answer is a generalized learning disability. This is diagnosed by an IQ of lower than 70. Other conditions are sometimes associated with learning difficulties, such as ASD, but you would expect to see other features of this in addition to a low IQ. Conditions such as ADHD can make it harder for young people to learn in standard settings, but again you would expect other behaviours to be present alongside the learning problem.

General feedback on 1–5: OHPsych 3rd edn → pp.624–5, 633, 637

→ NHS Choices—Encopresis: http://www.nhs.uk/conditions/encopresis/Pages/Introduction.aspx.

→ NHS Choices—Tics: http://www.nhs.uk/conditions/tics/pages/introduction.aspx.

→ Young Minds— What's worrying you? http://www.youngminds.org.uk/for_children_young_people/whats_worrying_you.

6. G ★★

The diagnosis in this case is oppositional defiant disorder which is a type of conduct disorder. According to NICE, conduct disorders are characterized by a repetitive and persistent pattern of antisocial, aggressive, or defiant conduct. Such behaviour is more severe than ordinary childish mischief or adolescent rebelliousness, and it goes beyond isolated antisocial acts. NICE guidance recommends group-based parent-training education programmes for children under 12 years old.

7. I ★★

According to NICE guidelines, adding fluoxetine (an SSRI) can be helpful if there has been no response to psychological therapy. If there is no response to a specific psychological therapy within four to six sessions, then review and consider alternative or additional psychological therapies for coexisting problems. Consider combining psychological therapy with fluoxetine (cautiously in younger children). If combined treatment is not effective within a further six sessions, review and consider more intensive psychological therapy.

8. B ★★

This young person is experiencing psychotic symptoms. It is important to assess how he is functioning at home and in school. Evidence suggests that untreated psychosis can be detrimental. Treatment is primarily pharmacological with antipsychotic medication.

9. J ★★

This young person may have an eating disorder. You do not know the extent of the weight loss of the BMI but have information that her hypothalamic-pituitary-adrenal axis is disturbed and this is one of the diagnostic features of anorexia nervosa. Assuming the young person is physically stable, treatment will consist of slow weight gain back to the normal range, following a meal plan, accompanied by family therapy.

10. H ★★

A behavioural intervention is the most appropriate in this case. Other forms of intervention can be adapted for use with those with learning disability, but behavioural interventions are the easiest to implement. Evidence shows that rewarding positive behaviours can increase their frequency and result in fewer negative behaviours.

General feedback on 6–10: OHPsych 3rd edn → pp.622–3, 651, 653

→ NICE Clinical Guideline 9—Eating disorders: http://publications. nice.org.uk/eating-disorders-cg9.

→ NICE Clinical Guideline 28—Depression in children and young peo- ple: http://www.nice.org.uk/CG28.

→ NICE Clinical Guideline 158—Antisocial behaviour and conduct disorders in children and young people: http://publications.nice.org. uk/antisocial-behaviour-and-conduct-disorders-in-children-and-yo ung-people-recognition-intervention-cg158.

Chapter 10

Psychiatry of old age

Clare Wadlow

This chapter of practice exam questions aims to put you, albeit briefly, in the seat of an old age psychiatrist dealing with important aspects of psychiatric disease in older adults. Our population is ageing and this, in addition to wider public understanding and earlier diagnoses of dementia, is leading to an increasing burden of disease. Furthermore it is acknowledged that the incidence of affective and psychotic disorders unexpectedly peaks again as we reach old age and can be devastating if not recognized and managed effectively.

The unique challenge of psychiatry of old age is the need for a sound grasp of general medicine and neurology to tackle unusual presentations of illness and possible multiple co-morbidities, in addition to a grounding in psychiatric theory. There remains a great need for lateral thinking, particularly in liaison work on the medical and surgical wards where delirium is rife and can masquerade as everything psychiatric. Within the specialty, true collaboration exists as allied health professionals and psychiatrists work together at problem solving to improve patients' quality of life beyond simply offering medication.

An understanding of the pathology, epidemiology, diagnosis, and treatment of mental illness and dementia in older adults is an essential skill for any doctor at the coalface. Working with older adults is incredibly rewarding and never stops being educational to the clinician. These patients and their carers will continue to challenge and impress you throughout your career.

As you manage to feel more confident with the facts, the practicalities and benefits of talking to and helping older adults become clearer. There is nothing that surpasses learning on the job, with many opportunities through attachments in psychiatry, GPs, ED, and geriatric wards. There are excellent resources available with regard to dementia, including NICE guidelines and the Alzheimer's Society website.

The aim of the following questions is to touch on a range of areas throughout the subject, taking us from first principles to practical application, through effective management, and support of older adults' mental health and wellbeing.

Clare Wadlow

QUESTIONS

Single Best Answers

1. A 75-year-old woman appears confused and forgetful for one week. She has told her family that her neighbours are stealing things from her fridge. She says she can see them hiding in the garden. She is labile in mood, distracted, and drowsy. Which is the *single* most appropriate first investigation? ★

A CT brain scan

B Dipstick mid-stream urine (MSU)

C FBC and differential white cell count (WCC)

D MSU culture and sensitivity

E Vitamin B₁₂ and folate serum level

2. A 73-year-old man has Alzheimer's dementia with an MMSE®-2™ of 24/30. He lives with his wife, although is largely independent, having only recently retired from teaching. He has never been lost or disorientated whilst away from home. He asks for advice about driving as his wife never learnt and relies on him. Which is the *single* most appropriate advice to give? ★

A He should arrange to undergo a driving assessment test

B He should inform the DVLA and his insurance company

C He should inform the DVLA who will retract his licence until he passes an assessment

D He should stop driving immediately

E His doctor should inform the DVLA on his behalf

3. A 78-year-old woman has recently been diagnosed with depression. She has started using St John's wort remedy to help improve her low mood. Which is the *single* most relevant advice to give her? ★

A It has not been shown to be particularly effective in depression

B It is not licensed for treating depression

C She cannot take it with her prescribed SSRI antidepressant

D She should not take it

E There may be significant interactions with her other medications

4. An 85-year-old woman is admitted to the ward with severe depression for six weeks. She is withdrawn and not sleeping well. She says she can't see the point of living, although she doesn't have any plans to actively end her life. Over the past four days she has stopped eating altogether and is drinking decreasing amounts of fluid. Which is the *single* most appropriate treatment at this stage? ★

A CBT and fluoxetine

B ECT

C Mirtazapine

D Nasogastric feeding

E Venlafaxine

5. A retired 76-year-old man with a UTI is septic and dehydrated. He has become aggressive and agitated, and is demanding to leave the ED as he says he has to go to work. Which is the *single* most appropriate management? ★

A Admit him to the medical ward under the Mental Capacity Act

B Ask him to complete a 'discharge against medical advice' form

C Detain him under Section 5(2) of the MHA

D Discharge him with a course of antibiotics with GP follow-up

E Organize an MHA assessment

6. An 85-year-old man has disinhibition, personality change, and minor cognitive deficits, according to his sister. A provisional diagnosis of FTD is made. Which *single* feature is most likely to support this diagnosis? ★

A Apathy

B Hallucinations

C Patient's age

D Patient's gender

E Widespread atrophic changes on CT brain scan

7. A 79-year-old man has short-term memory loss, non-troublesome visual hallucinations, and some stiffness and tremor for nine months. His MMSE®-2™ score is 23/30. Which is the *single* most appropriate medication to slow cognitive decline? ★★

A Donepezil

B Galantamine

C Levodopa

D Memantine

E Rivastigmine

8. A 74-year-old woman becomes increasingly confused over a period of six months. Before a formal diagnosis could be made, she died of a heart attack. A provisional diagnosis of Alzheimer's dementia was made, and her daughter would like to know if this was the case. She agrees to an autopsy. Which *single* neuropathological finding would be most likely to confirm this diagnosis? ★★

A Cytoplasmic inclusion bodies

B Extracellular neurofibrillary tangles

C Extracellular senile plaques

D Knife-edge atrophy

E Pick's bodies

9. An 83-year-old woman with Alzheimer's dementia who has recently started taking donepezil is reviewed in the memory clinic. Which is the *single* most appropriate observation to review? ★★

A Abbreviated mental test score

B Blood pressure

C Geriatric Depression Scale

D Pulse

E Respiratory rate

10. A 67-year-old woman has been prescribed memantine to treat her dementia. Her son, a biochemist, asks which group of receptors this medication is primarily active at. Which is the *single* most appropriate answer to give? ★★

A Cholinergic

B Dopaminergic

C Glutamatergic

D Muscarinic

E Serotonergic

11. A 75-year-old man has been diagnosed with Lewy body dementia in memory clinic. Which *single* symptom or sign most strongly indicates this diagnosis? ★★★

A Falls and syncope

B Rapid eye movement (REM) sleep disorder

C Severe neuroleptic sensitivity

D Visual hallucinations

E Word-finding difficulties

12. An 83-year-old woman with severe Alzheimer's dementia lives in a nursing home. Staff report that she is stable and presents no problems to them. Her MMSE®-2™ score is 9/30. Her list of medications is being reviewed. Which *single* medication is the most appropriate to stop first? ★★★

A Co-codamol 8/500 PRN maximum qds

B Donepezil 10 mg once daily

C Olanzapine 5 mg at night

D Simvastatin 20 mg at night

E Temazepam 10 mg at night as needed

13. A 74-year-old man feels tired during the day but doesn't know why. His wife says he is up overnight fighting with the bed sheets and at these times tells her he can see snakes. They have put padding on the bedside table to prevent injury. Which is the *single* most likely diagnosis? ★★★★

A Alzheimer's dementia

B Delirium

C Harmful use of alcohol

D Psychosis

E REM sleep disorder

14. A 78-year-old man has accrued rental arrears for the past 12 months as he now firmly believes that he owns his flat, despite being a renting council tenant for many years. Which *single* additional feature in his history would increase his risk of a late-onset psychotic episode? ★★★★

A Family history of Alzheimer's dementia

B Hearing impairment

C Living with a dependent partner

D Male gender

E Vascular disease

Extended Matching Questions

Dementia diagnoses

For each scenario, choose the *single* most likely diagnosis from the list below. Each option may be used once, more than once, or not at all. ★

A Alcoholic amnesic syndrome

B Alzheimer's dementia

C Delirium

D Dementia in Parkinson's disease

E FTD

F Lewy body dementia

G Normal pressure hydrocephalus

H Pseudodementia

I Semantic dementia

J Vascular dementia

1. An 85-year-old woman has gradually worsening memory problems for 12 months. She left her keys in the door twice, is less interested in bridge nights, and stopped going to choir six months ago. She got lost on her way home last week. She experiences some word-finding difficulties.

2. A 65-year-old man is noted to be more irritable by his wife. He has started swearing in public, and eats more sweet foods and drinks more alcohol. He has been asked to retire from work as his performance is poor. Sometimes he says the wrong word when speaking.

3. An 85-year-old man has been unsteady on his feet since a fall six months ago. His family have noticed he had a sudden deterioration in his short-term memory and he has become more emotional. The memory has neither worsened nor improved since the fall.

4. A 67-year-old woman is worried about memory loss. She reports being unable to concentrate or sleep well. She feels her memory is worse in the mornings. She answers 'I don't know' to many questions on the MMSE®-2™, particularly scoring poorly on attention and recall tasks.

5. A 71-year-old man with Parkinson's disease for three years has more recently been seeing a small, black cat running around the house in the evenings, although his wife cannot see it. At times he is disorientated and muddled and can be quite repetitive. His wife thinks his symptoms have been gradually getting worse.

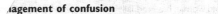
nagement of confusion

For each of the psychiatry of old age liaison scenarios described, choose the *single* best first step to manage the situation from the list below. Each option may be used once, more than once, or not at all. ★★★

A Admit to psychiatry ward
B Chlordiazepoxide 20 mg four times daily
C Diazepam 5 mg PRN
D Lithium 200 mg twice daily
E Mirtazapine 15 mg at night
F Nurse in a well-lit, quiet side room
G Quetiapine 25 mg at night
H Risperidone 0.5 mg at night
I Venlafaxine XL 75 mg once daily
J Watchful waiting

6. A 69-year-old woman becomes acutely disturbed on the ward three days after a knee replacement operation. She is trying to leave the ward as she says she can see creatures crawling on the floor. She is tremulous and hypertensive.

7. A 74-year-old man was admitted to a medical ward as he was found confused and wandering. Each evening he becomes upset with staff as he feels threatened. He has also talked about seeing babies on the ward and at times asks why he is in a nursery.

8. An 84-year-old woman has been in hospital for six weeks with a severe community-acquired pneumonia. She is almost ready for discharge but has stopped eating and is sending the physiotherapist away. Staff report that she seems withdrawn and tearful and is not sleeping well.

9. A 72-year-old woman with Parkinson's disease for some years is admitted following a fall when walking to buy food for people who had come into her lounge. A friend says there was no-one there and explains that the patient often talks to people who are not present. The patient tells you that she feels exhausted having to cater for so many people in her house and that they continue to bother her on the ward.

10. A 91-year-old man is admitted to a medical ward following a collapse in the street. Physical examination and blood and urine screens have revealed no abnormalities. He is very talkative and agitated, not sleeping, and eating little. He has tried to leave as he says he must get to work on a new project. His family are worried about him as he has remortgaged the house and on two occasions pushed his elderly wife over.

ANSWERS

Single Best Answers

1. B ★   OHPsych 3rd edn → pp.790–2

UTIs are a very common cause of delirium in the elderly. Dipstick urinanalysis is an easy and useful first test in any setting (B).

A CT brain scan (A) is an important part of a full dementia screen, especially if there are any atypical features; e.g. short history or sudden decline, younger age at onset of symptoms, focal neurological signs. However, in this case, because of the short onset of symptoms, visual hallucinations, and associated drowsiness, the more likely diagnosis in this patient is delirium. Remember, for a diagnosis of dementia you need a history of symptoms for at least six months in clear consciousness.

FBC is an important part of the dementia screen. The differential WCC (C) might help point towards a diagnosis of delirium, although it is not as quick or specific a result as a urine dipstick.

MSU culture and sensitivity (D) would be an important next step if the dipstick is positive.

Testing vitamin B_{12} and folate (E) is an essential part of a dementia screen, as low levels of either can masquerade as dementia or exacerbate an existing dementia. However, this appears to be a presentation of delerium and this would not be the best immediate investigation.

→ Lindesay J (2007). Delirium. In: M Gelder, J Lopéz-Ibor, N Andreasen (eds) *New Oxford Textbook of Psychiatry*, 2nd edn. Oxford University Press, Oxford.

→ NICE Clinical Guideline 103—Delirium: http://www.nice.org.uk/cg103.

2. B ★   OHPsych 3rd edn → pp.136–7

The man should be advised to inform both the DVLA and his insurance company (B). The DVLA would then ask for consent to contact his GP or specialist for medical information and based on this may ask him to undertake a driving assessment. Then he may be issued with a licence for a shorter period and need regular reassessments, or he may be asked to stop driving.

(A) is partly correct but he should be advised to inform the DVLA and his insurance company. He may wish to undergo an assessment for his own information and reassurance or the DVLA may ask him to.

He should inform the DVLA but they will not automatically retract his licence (C). He may have to complete a driving assessment.

Stopping driving immediately (D) may be advisable if the doctor is very worried about the patient's driving safety, but based on the history given in this question, there is no evidence to suggest he needs to be told to stop driving immediately.

That his doctor should inform the DVLA on his behalf (E) is not the best initial piece of advice. However, if a patient refuses to contact the DVLA, a doctor may do this without the patient's consent if the doctor is concerned for the safety of that person or other road users. If a doctor does decide to breach confidentiality and inform the DVLA the doctor has a professional duty to try to inform the patient of their intentions, and should confirm in writing once this disclosure has been made.

→ Alzheimer's Society—Driving and dementia: http://alzheimers.org.uk/site/scripts/documents_info.php?documentID=144.

3. E ★   OHPsych 3rd edn → p.276

The most important thing a patient should know about St John's wort is that there may be significant interactions with other medications (E). It induces the cytochrome P450 enzyme and therefore can cause significant interactions with important medications such as warfarin, antiretrovirals, and the contraceptive pill.

Evidence shows that St John's wort could be effective in the treatment of mild or moderate depression but there is less evidence for its use in severe depression (A).

Most preparations are not licensed in this country (B). It is used more in some other countries, e.g. Germany.

It is not absolutely contraindicated with SSRIs (C).

Helping the patient to make an informed decision is more professional and respectful than forbidding her to take the remedy (D). Patients will of course ultimately do what they think is best for them, and this approach could significantly jeopardize the doctor–patient relationship.

4. B ★   OHPsych 3rd edn → pp.282–7

ECT (B) is an effective, fast, and relatively safe treatment for an elderly patient with severe depression. The information that this patient is not eating and is drinking little makes this a very urgent case and she needs treatment that will work quickly. ECT is therefore the best option in this case. Thankfully there are very few absolute contraindications and her age certainly does not exclude her from receiving this potentially life-saving therapy.

CBT and fluoxetine (A) are good treatments for depression and potentiate each other if used together. However, this patient does not appear to be well enough to respond to psychological interventions.

Mirtazapine (C) is a good antidepressant for those patients who are not eating or sleeping well, particularly as the side-effect profile can therefore be beneficial. However, in this urgent case, oral medication is unlikely to work quickly enough.

Nasogastric feeding (D) may be needed if she does not improve, but it will not treat the depression itself.

Venlafaxine (E) is a good antidepressant for those patients who have not responded to adequate trials of SSRIs, but in this urgent case it is unlikely to work quickly enough.

→ O'Connor DW (2008). Electroconvulsive therapy. In: R Jacoby, C Oppenheimer, T Dening, A Thomas (eds) *Oxford Textbook of Old Age Psychiatry*, 4th edn, p.201. Oxford University Press, Oxford.

5. A ★　　　　　OHPsych 3rd edn → pp.794–5

The most appropriate management would be to admit this man to the medical ward under the Mental Capacity Act (A). He may well be delirious. It is very unlikely that he has capacity to decide to leave hospital. The Mental Capacity Act has replaced what was known as 'common law' and allows treatment of medical conditions against a patient's wishes if in their best interests and in a least restrictive format if they are assessed to lack capacity concerning treatment decisions.

Although sometimes a tempting option in a busy ED, this patient is septic, elderly, and unlikely to be making clear decisions or have the capacity to decide to go home. He would be a great risk if allowed to leave; therefore asking him to complete a 'discharge against medical advice' form is a line of action that would be unsafe and negligent (B).

Section 5(2) of the MHA allows for already admitted patients to be detained in hospital until a full MHA assessment can be arranged, for a maximum of 72 hours. It cannot be used for patients in an ED as they are not yet admitted; therefore (C) is not the right answer. It is also not appropriate in this case as the patient is likely to lack capacity due to physical illness, and therefore the Mental Capacity Act is the relevant legislation to refer to.

Although prescribing antibiotics to take at home is attempting to treat the underlying cause of this man's presentation, it would be unsafe to assume that he will understand and be compliant with this. He may well deteriorate and would certainly be a risk to himself if allowed to leave at this point (D).

This patient would be best served by the Mental Capacity Act as the MHA (E) only allows for treatment of mental illnesses, not physical ones.

→ Mental Capacity Act Legislation 2005: http://www.legislation.gov.uk/ukpga/2005/9/contents.

6. A ★　　　　　OHPsych 3rd edn → pp.142–3

Significant apathy (A) and withdrawn behaviour is often a feature of FTD. Patients may present with personality change, disinhibition, and impulsivity before any cognitive deficits emerge. They may be getting into trouble at work or within families for their strange behaviour. They may be wrongly diagnosed with depression or other psychiatric conditions.

Hallucinations (B) are not particularly common in FTD. However, all dementia patients are susceptible to superimposed delirium.

Patients with FTD tend to present at an earlier age, typically 45–60 years old (C).

Although men are more likely to develop FTD, this feature is not the most suggestive of this diagnosis (D).

Involutional or atrophic changes may be seen in any ageing brain (E). They are often seen in those with Alzheimer's dementia to a more severe extent. If widespread, they would not be helpful to diagnose FTD. If the changes are more evident in the frontal and temporal lobes this may contribute to a diagnosis of FTD.

→ Pasquier F, Deramecourt V, Lebert F (2008). Clinical aspects of dementia: frontotemporal dementia. In: R Jacoby, C Oppenheimer, T Dening, A Thomas (eds) *Oxford Textbook of Old Age Psychiatry*, 4th edn, pp.462–3. Oxford University Press, Oxford.

7. E ★★   OHPsych 3rd edn → pp.138–9

Rivastigmine (*Exelon*™) (E) has the biggest body of evidence currently for use in Lewy body dementia.

Donepezil (*Aricept*™) (A) is an acetylcholinesterase inhibitor prescribed most readily for patients with Alzheimer's dementia. It would be a reasonable choice but is not the first option as this patient's symptoms point to a diagnosis of Lewy body dementia.

Galantamine (*Reminyl*™) (B) is another acetylcholinesterase inhibitor that can be used for dementia. It is more expensive than donepezil and rivastigmine and tends to be used less as a first-line treatment.

Levodopa (C) would primarily be used to treat the motor symptoms of Parkinson's and has no significant effects on memory.

Memantine (*Ebixor*™) (D) is recommended by NICE to be used to treat moderate to severe dementia. It may also be used in patients who cannot tolerate other antidementia medication due to cardiac arrhythmias as it is a safer option.

→ NICE Technology Appraisal TA217—Donepezil, galantamine, rivastigmine and memantine for the treatment of Alzheimer's disease: http://www.nice.org.uk/guidance/index.jsp?action=byID&o=13419.

8. C ★★   OHPsych 3rd edn → pp.134–5

Extracellular senile plaques (C) are found in Alzheimer's dementia. They can also be found in the normal ageing brain to some extent. Their main component is amyloid, formed by abnormal metabolism of a larger amino acid.

Inclusion bodies are nuclear or cytoplasmic aggregates of stainable substances, usually proteins. Cytoplasmic inclusion bodies (A) are found with certain viral infections, such as rabies and smallpox whereas neuronal inclusion bodies are found in diseases like Parkinson's disease and Lewy body dementia.

In Alzheimer's disease there are intracellular neurofibrillary tangles, not extracellular (B). These are abnormal structures that accumulate inside neurons, made principally of hyperphosphorylated tau proteins.

Knife-edge atrophy (D) refers to the extreme and global thinning of the gyri of the cerebral cortex seen in the frontal and temporal lobes in Pick's disease.

Pick's bodies (E) are also intracellular neurofibrillary tangles composed of abnormal tau proteins but they differ from those found in Alzheimer's disease as they stain differently and are more straight and fibrous. Those in Alzheimer's are paired and coiled.

→ Nagy Z, Hubbard P (2008). Neuropathology. In: R Jacoby, C Oppenheimer, T Dening, A Thomas (eds) *Oxford Textbook of Old Age Psychiatry*, 4th edn. Oxford University Press, Oxford.

9. **D** ★★ OHPsych 3rd edn → pp.138–9

Donepezil and other acetylcholinesterase inhibitors have been shown in clinical trials to slow the heart rate by on average 1–2 bpm (D). They may also increase the heart rate interval. If a patient has first-degree heart block, this medication may cause arrhythmia, syncope, and collapse. It is good practice to obtain an ECG prior to prescribing the medication and to monitor a patient's pulse during treatment.

Abbreviated mental test scores (A), usually the MMSE®-2™, are used to monitor progress. This should be recorded prior to starting medication, and then at approximately six-monthly intervals, as well as measures of functioning and behaviour.

BP (B) is not known to be significantly impacted by donepezil.

The Geriatric Depression Scale (C) would be a useful tool if concerns about low mood were present. It is not routinely used in monitoring donepezil in dementia.

Respiratory rate is not known to be affected by these medications (E).

→ Wilcock G (2008). Clinical aspects of dementia: specific pharmacological treatments for Alzheimer's disease. In: R Jacoby, C Oppenheimer, T Dening, A Thomas (eds) *Oxford Textbook of Old Age Psychiatry*, 4th edn, p.485. Oxford University Press, Oxford.

→ Bordier P, Garrigue S, Lanusse S, *et al.* (2006). Cardiovascular effects and risk of syncope related to donepezil in patients with Alzheimer's disease. *CNS Drugs*, **20** (5), 411–17.

10. **C** ★★ OHPsych 3rd edn → pp.132–3

Glutamatergic (C) is the correct answer. Memantine is an antagonist at the glutamatergic NMDA receptors.

Memantine is thought to have some activity on cholinergic receptors (A) but its significance is unclear. The other antidementia medications (donepezil and rivastigmine) are acetylcholinesterase inhibitors, boosting the amount of acetylcholine available in the brain.

Again, memantine is thought to have some activity at dopaminergic receptors (B) but it is not the main action thought to be responsible for its benefits. It is believed that antipsychotic medications achieve their positive effects on psychotic symptoms by blocking these receptors.

Muscarinic receptors (D) are a type of cholinergic receptor. Acetylcholine acts here and therefore these are more related to the action of the other antidementia medications.

The clinical significance of memantine's antagonistic action at the serotonergic receptors (E) is unknown.

→ Wilcock G (2008). Clinical aspects of dementia: specific pharmaco-logical treatments for Alzheimer's disease. In: R Jacoby, C Oppenheimer, T Dening, A Thomas (eds) *Oxford Textbook of Old Age Psychiatry*, 4th edn, p.486. Oxford University Press, Oxford.

11. D ★★★   OHPsych 3rd edn → pp.140–1

Visual hallucinations (D) are one of the three core features of Lewy body dementia: (1) visual hallucinations, typically well formed and not particularly distressing; (2) fluctuating cognition with variations in atten-tion and alertness; and (3) spontaneous features of Parkinson's disease (present for less than a year before cognitive problems).

Falls and syncope (A) often are a feature of the presentation of Lewy body dementia but are not very specific for the diagnosis. Falls often occur because the patient's gait and balance are affected by the motor symptoms of Parkinson's.

REM sleep disorder (B) is a common symptom of Lewy body demen-tia which can be very tricky to manage. Patients complain of very vivid dreams and relatives notice disturbed sleep and at times disorientation and wandering at night with associated odd behaviours. However, this is not one of the core symptoms and so this is not the strongest indicator of the diagnosis.

Severe neuroleptic sensitivity (C) refers to the common reaction these patients can have to any antipsychotic medication. They can become acutely confused, experience severe extrapyramidal symptoms, and have an increased mortality rate.

Word-finding difficulties (E) are often a presenting feature of any demen-tia and do not indicate Lewy body dementia in particular.

→ McKeith TG, Dickson DW, Lowe J, *et al.* and the DLB Consortium (2005). Diagnosis and management of dementia with Lewy bodies. *Neurology*, **65** (12), 1863–72.

12. C ★★★   OHPsych 3rd edn → pp.138–9

Antipsychotics in dementia have been shown to carry a substantial risk of morbidity and mortality, e.g. increased risk of stroke. It is best to avoid their use completely. However, if clinically necessary they need frequent review with an aim to stop as soon as possible. Olanzapine (C) especially is best avoided all together and therefore this would be the most urgent medication to try to stop.

Codeine-based medications can cause constipation and other side-effects in the elderly and are therefore generally best avoided (A). It is best to manage pain with the lowest possible strength but is not imperative to stop this if needed.

NICE guidelines continue to recommend that donepezil and related medications are discontinued when a patient's dementia becomes severe (B). However, there is recent evidence to suggest that a per-son's behaviour and memory deficit may significantly deteriorate if it is stopped. Many clinicians choose to continue the medication as this is often the family's wishes. Additionally it is now available off-label and therefore much less costly than it used to be.

It is reasonable in severe dementia to try to stop all non-essential medication. However, if a person is tolerating their simvastatin (D), this will reduce the vascular risk burden of disease and thus potential slow progression of cognitive deficit.

Benzodiazepines such as temazepam (E) are best used only for short-term treatments, if at all. However, they are thought to be safer than antipsychotics in dementia.

→ Thomas A (2008). Clinical aspects of dementia: Alzheimer's disease. In: R Jacoby, C Oppenheimer, T Dening, A Thomas (eds) *Oxford Textbook of Old Age Psychiatry*, 4th edn, pp.425–42. Oxford University Press, Oxford.

---

13. E ★★★★   OHPsych 3rd edn → p.446

This presentation is likely to be REM sleep disorder (E). People can injure themselves and others without being awake during very vivid dreams when normally atonic muscles become active during REM, dream sleep. It can be a presentation of a Lewy body dementia. Treatment is often clonazepam or other sedatives. It is also important to consider the risk of injury to the patient and their bed partner.

People with Alzheimer's dementia (A) do often report sleep disturbance. It is likely that they are more confused in the evenings. A concern is that they may become disorientated overnight and wander. If the man in the scenario above also had other features of dementia, the diagnosis may well be Lewy body dementia.

Delirium (B) can present with visual hallucinations and dreams that seem very vivid and merge with reality. There will usually be other features present such as a variable level of consciousness, confusion, and distractibility. It is unlikely to only occur at night.

Elderly people are just as susceptible to harmful alcohol use (C) as younger adults, if not more so. Visual hallucinations can be signs of a withdrawal, but this is more likely to occur some days after suddenly stopping or reducing alcohol intake.

True psychosis (D) would have a different flavour from this presentation. There would more likely be auditory hallucinations and delusional ideas present or other disorders of thought. Again, these would normally be pervasive and not just at night.

→ Mosimann UP, Boeve BF (2008). In: R Jacoby, C Oppenheimer, T Dening, A Thomas (eds) *Oxford Textbook of Old Age Psychiatry*, 4th edn, pp.681–2. Oxford University Press, Oxford.

---

14. B ★★★★   OHPsych 3rd edn → pp.522–3

Sensory impairment (B) is a risk factor for late-onset psychosis; it is thought to add to social isolation. Not having family or friends to allow social interaction and support is a significant risk factor for these episodes.

Family history of psychotic symptoms may be a risk factor for this condition, but a history of dementia is more relevant for patients presenting with cognitive deficits (A).

Living with a dependent partner (C) would be a risk factor more relevant for mood or neurotic disorders.

There is actually a female preponderance for later-onset schizophrenia and paraphrenias, not male (D).

Vascular disease is a significant risk factor in the dementias (E).

→ Howard R (2008). Late onset schizophrenia and very late onset schizophrenia-like psychosis. In: R Jacoby, C Oppenheimer, T Dening, A Thomas (eds) *Oxford Textbook of Old Age Psychiatry*, 4th edn, pp.617–26. Oxford University Press, Oxford.

Extended Matching Questions

1. B ★

This is a typical presentation of Alzheimer's dementia: gradual deterioration in short-term memory, affecting functioning. There is often associated apathy and decreased interest in activities previously enjoyed. Word-finding difficulties are common.

2. E ★

Frontotemporal dementia tends to present in a younger age group than Alzheimer's or vascular dementia. Memory deficits are often present at a later stage. Personality changes, disinhibition, and other frontal lobe symptoms are seen first. Difficulties with the meaning of language may be present, though speech is normally fluent.

3. J ★

It is possible that the fall was a stroke, and a step-wise deterioration in memory and functioning is seen. It is common for patients with vascular dementia to develop emotional lability. He may have focal neurological deficits, and vascular changes would be seen on a CT brain scan.

4. H ★

This relatively young patient is typical of someone who actually has a predominant mood disorder that is affecting their memory. She herself is worried about her memory which follows the pattern of diurnal mood variation. In true dementias, patients often don't notice their cognitive deficit and are often more confused at night (known as 'sundowning'). Patients with depression will often say they do not know the answers on the MMSE®-2™ in contrast to those with dementia who are more likely to guess wrong answers.

5. D ★

Cognitive decline, visual hallucinations, and parkinsonian symptoms are also features of Lewy body dementia, but as this patient has had the motor symptoms of Parkinson's disease for more than one year, it would be named a Parkinson's dementia.

General feedback on 1–5: OHPsych 3rd edn → pp.132–50

6. B ★★★

This woman has a sudden-onset post-operative delirium. It is about the right length of time for alcohol withdrawal to develop. Her physical state and hypertension are pointing towards this diagnosis. She may also have nystagmus and tachycardia. A full alcohol history, ideally confirmed by a collateral history, would be essential. Small animal or insect visual hallucinations are typical of this group of patients. This patient could do much damage to her new knee replacement and could also be developing Wernicke's encephalopathy. She needs urgent management with a chlordiazepoxide reducing regimen and parenteral thiamine. She will need regular observation and possibly 1:1 nursing as well.

7. F ★★★

This is an extremely common referral. The patient is showing signs of an acute confusion or delirium. Much investigation needs to be done to discover the cause, including a full delirium screen and collateral history to establish his baseline functioning and cognition. When the cause of confusion is identified the best step is to treat this. Until then, avoiding antipsychotics or sedation if possible is recommended, although he may need these if he becomes distressed. Simple measures such as a calmer, quieter environment and frequent reorientation and explanation may help ameliorate his symptoms.

8. E ★★★

This woman has symptoms of depression, although a full history and MSE are needed to confirm this. A sensible first step would be to trial an antidepressant. Given that her pattern of symptoms includes poor sleep and appetite, mirtazapine is a good first-line treatment as its side-effects may help improve these. Venlafaxine is also an option but not often used first line and has a less beneficial side-effect profile in this case.

9. G ★★★

Unfortunately Parkinson's disease and its treatments can cause psychosis which is difficult to treat without worsening the movement disorder. Quetiapine is currently the antipsychotic of choice in patients who also have Parkinson's as it has been shown to be helpful for psychosis with fewest detrimental side-effects. Quetiapine is therefore a better choice in this case than risperidone which is often used as a first-line treatment for psychosis in other older patients.

10. A ★★★

With no physical cause found for this man's symptoms, it seems likely that he may be experiencing mania. There are significant risk factors present in his history to himself (wandering, impulsivity, poor appetite) and to others (mortgaging the house, aggression towards his wife). Therefore it would be best to assess and treat him further on a psychiatry inpatient ward, until his risk can be contained and support continued in the community.

General feedback on 6–10: OHPsych 3rd edn → pp.988, 990–1

→ Hogg J (2008). Delirium. In: R Jacoby, C Oppenheimer, T Dening, A Thomas (eds) *Oxford Textbook of Old Age Psychiatry*, 4th edn, pp.505–17. Oxford University Press, Oxford.

Learning disability

Maggie McGurgan and Holly Greer

Intellectual disability is defined by the World Health Organization (WHO) as: 'a significantly reduced ability to understand new or complex information and to learn and apply new skills (impaired intelligence) resulting in a reduced ability to cope independently (impaired social functioning)', and begins before adulthood, with a lasting effect on development.

People with an intellectual disability can develop any of the mental illnesses common to the general population; however, they are up to three times more likely to develop a mental illness. This predisposition to psychiatric illness can occur due to a variety of reasons, including associated genetic syndromes, brain injury, and sensory impairments. People with an intellectual disability are also more likely to have negative psychosocial experiences, such as deprivation, abuse, separation/loss events, low self-esteem, and financial disadvantage, and consequently the ensuing effects of these can affect their mental health.

The psychiatric assessment of a person with an intellectual disability broadly covers the same as that of the general population; however, a different approach at times is needed to adapt to the individual's communication skills. It may be necessary to complete history taking from a family member or carer, and an MSE may even have to be completed solely on observable behaviours. It is also more pertinent to focus on any co-existing medical conditions, such as epilepsy which is present in 25–30% of people with an intellectual disability.

The WHO states that the true prevalence of intellectual disability is close to 3%. The vast majority of these people (85%) have mild intellectual disability defined as an IQ of 50–69 points. Many of these people can and do access mainstream services (with or without additional support). In whichever service you work, doctors and medical students will encounter people with intellectual disabilities, and an awareness of their needs is essential.

Maggie McGurgan and Holly Greer

QUESTIONS

Single Best Answers

1. A 42-year-old man with Down's syndrome has recent-onset brief episodes of shaking, confusion, and unusual behaviour, followed by prolonged somnolence. Which is the *single* most likely cause of these episodes? ★

A BPAD

B Challenging behaviour

C Depression

D Epilepsy related to dementia

E Transient ischaemic attacks

2. A six-year-old boy has a learning disability thought to be of genetic origin as he has suggestive facial features including prominent epicanthic folds. Chromosomal blood investigations have been performed to see if a specific cause can be identified. A student nurse at clinic asks what the most likely chromosomal cause of his learning disability is. Which is the *single* most likely diagnosis? ★

A Cri du chat syndrome

B Down's syndrome

C Klinefelter's syndrome

D Prader–Willi syndrome

E Turner's syndrome

3. The father of a six-year-old girl with an IQ of 55 is concerned that she has autism as he has read that this is often co-morbid with learning disability. Which *single* characteristic feature is most associated with this condition? ★

A Abnormalities in social relatedness, communication, and behaviours

B Intense sensory responsiveness

C Neurological abnormalities including seizures and motor tics

D Restricted and stereotyped interests

E Savant peaks of remarkable ability

4. A 24-year-old man with learning disability is being assessed in an outpatient clinic for the first time. Which is the *single* most important part of this assessment process? ★

A Collateral history from the patient's carer

B Complete MSE

C Considering the communication needs of the patient

D Developmental history

E Physical examination of the patient

5. A 38-year-old man with moderate learning disability is admitted from a residential home to a medical ward due to deteriorating function. No medical cause has been found to explain this. The medical team have requested a psychiatric assessment. Despite best efforts it is hard to get information from him. Which is the *single* most appropriate source of collateral history in this circumstance? ★

A GP

B Girlfriend

C Medical ward staff

D Parents

E Residential home staff

6. A 43-year-old man has both epilepsy and learning disability. His sister asks if he is simply unlucky to have two separate problems or if they are connected. She is told that he is in the IQ subgroup known to have the highest association with epilepsy. Which *single* IQ range is he likely to be in? ★★

A IQ < 20

B IQ 20–34

C IQ 35–49

D IQ 50–69

E IQ 70–94

7. A 14-year-old adolescent has marked behavioural and interpersonal difficulties. He has a moderate learning disability, mild ASD, and complex attachment problems. Which *single* psychological therapy is the most appropriate treatment for him? ★★

A CBT

B Family therapy

C Narrative therapy

D Not appropriate for any form of psychological therapy

E Psychoanalytic psychotherapy

8. A 35-year-old man with a mild learning disability and epilepsy has a moderate–severe depressive episode. His is taking carbamazepine 400 mg BD, and has been referred for CBT. Which is the *single* most appropriate treatment option? ★★★

A Start antidepressant at half normal initiation dose. Titrate up at half recommended titration rate

B Start antidepressant at normal initiation dose. Titrate up at normal titration rate

C Start antidepressant at normal initiation dose. Titrate up rapidly

D Start antidepressant at normal initiation dose with benzodiazepine. Titrate up antidepressant rapidly

E Start antidepressant at normal initiation dose with low-dose antipsychotic. Titrate up antidepressant rapidly

Extended Matching Questions

Extended Matching Questions

Learning disability diagnoses

For each scenario below, choose the *single* most likely cause of learning disability from the list of options. Each option may be used once, more than once, or not at all. ★★

A Down's syndrome

B Fragile X syndrome

C Klinefelter's syndrome

D Phenylketonuria

E Prader–Willi syndrome

F Rett syndrome

G Sotos syndrome

H Trisomy X

I Tuberous sclerosis (TS) complex

J Turner's syndrome

1. A 22-year-old woman has short stature, prominent epicanthic folds, low-set ears, and a protruding tongue. Her speech is difficult to understand. Her carer describes her as having typical biological features of depression.

2. A 14-year-old adolescent has short stature, marked central obesity, and small hands and feet. His parents are finding it difficult to manage his behavioural outbursts, often related to seeking food.

3. A 24-year-old man has difficulties coping with changes to his routine and displays restlessness and ritualistic behaviours. He has a long narrow face, large head and ears, and does not make eye contact.

4. A newborn baby is experiencing recurrent seizures. She was born in a squat and her mother is a homeless Eastern European asylum seeker with no antenatal or post-natal care. The baby has very fair skin, a small head, and is failing to thrive. There is a musty odour to her urine.

5. A four-year-old boy has seizures, physically aggressive behaviour, and features of autism. He has red facial papules, depigmented skin patches, numerous light brown skin patches of varying sizes, and flesh-coloured papules at his nail beds.

Congenital causes of learning disability

Certain causes of learning disability have particular associations with psychiatric problems. For each of the psychiatric presentations below, choose the *single* most likely associated cause of learning disability from the list of options. Each option may be used once, more than once, or not at all. ★★★★

A Congenital syphilis

B Down's syndrome

C Fetal alcohol syndrome

D Fragile X syndrome

E Hunter syndrome

F Lesch–Nyhan syndrome

G Neonatal hypoxic brain injury

H Prader–Willi syndrome

I Sturge–Weber syndrome

J Velo-cardio-facial syndrome (VCFS)

6. A 31-year-old man with learning difficulties appears to be responding to visual and auditory hallucinations.

7. A 28-year-old woman with learning difficulties is experiencing early morning wakening, reduced motivation for favoured activities, loss of appetite, weight loss, and diurnal variation of mood.

8. A 12-year-old boy with learning difficulties is engaging in frequent and severe self-injurious behaviours including biting and head banging.

9. A 27-year-old man with learning difficulties is very rigid and inflexible regarding his daily activities and routines. He has been found to hoard objects and to have obsessional tendencies about his property and environment.

10. A 15-year-old adolescent with learning difficulties has marked difficulties with social interaction and prefers not to make eye contact. He is uncomfortable engaging in conversation.

ANSWERS

Single Best Answers

1. D ★   OHPsych 3rd edn → pp.744–5

People with Down's syndrome are at very high risk of developing Alzheimer-type dementia as they advance in years. Epilepsy as a marker for this onset is quite a common feature (D).

BPAD (A) typically presents with a history of clear, lengthy episodes of mood elevation or depression. This would also be the case for patients with a learning disability, although the presentation may be more subtle and more difficult to distinguish from other behaviours.

Challenging behaviour (B) (or more properly labelled 'behaviour which is experienced as challenging') is a frequent issue amongst patients with learning disabilities. One must never assume that it is solely related to the cause of the learning disability. Physical and mental illnesses as well as environmental and social difficulties should be considered.

Depression (C) in a person with a learning disability will generally show the same biological features as in the general population. The presentation may be more subtle or indeed more exaggerated and can be difficult to distinguish from other behaviours.

Transient ischaemic attacks (E) will generally present in their typical fashion in a person with a learning disability. The difficulty can be when carers or medical staff attribute these typical signs and symptoms to other issues.

→ Menéndez M (2005). Down syndrome, Alzheimer's disease and seizures. *Brain and Development*, **27** (4), 246–52.

→ Prasher V (2006). *Down's Syndrome and Alzheimer's Disease—Biological Correlates*, Chapter 6. Radcliffe Health, Oxford.

2. B ★   OHPsych 3rd edn → pp.746–7

Down's syndrome (B) is the commonest chromosomal cause of learning disability. It occurs as full trisomy 21 in 95% of cases, Robertsonian translocation is the cause in about 5%, and mosaicism in 2–5%.

Intellectual disability is a very common symptom in Cri du Chat syndrome (A). The severity depends on how much of the fifth chromosome's petit arm is deleted.

Intellect is not normally affected in people with Klinefelter's syndrome (C), but there may be delays in motor skills and language development among affected males.

Most people with Prader–Willi syndrome (D) have mild intellectual disabilities.

The majority of females with Turner's syndrome (E) have normal intelligence. A small proportion may have a learning disability.

→ Cornish K, Bramble D (2002). Cri du chat syndrome: genotype–phenotype correlations and recommendations for clinical management. *Development Medicine and Child Neurology*, **44** (7), 494–7.

→ Debenham L (2012). *Down's syndrome*. About Learning Disabilities: http://www.aboutlearningdisabilities.co.uk/downs-syndrome.html.

→ Understanding Intellectual Disability and Health: http://www.intellectualdisability.info/.

3. A ★   OHPysch 3rd edn → pp.630–1

The classical triad of features of autism includes abnormalities in social relatedness, communication, and behaviours (A). The onset of these is before three years of age, although parents often notice signs within the first two years of life.

Intense sensory responsiveness (B) is commonly seen in ASD but is not part of the classic autism triad.

Epilepsy is the most common medical condition occurring in those with ASD, but seizures or tics are not necessary to make the diagnosis (C).

Having restricted and stereotyped interests (D) is very commonly seen in autism and ASD but is not one of the cardinal features.

Savant syndrome describes the condition when people with significant mental difficulties possess exceptional skills in specific areas, far beyond what is considered normal, e.g. memory or calculation abilities. Although 50% of savants are thought to have autism, 'savant skills' are not a common finding in people with autism (E).

4. C ★   OHPsych 3rd edn → pp.738–9

Where communication is optimized and the patient can give their own history (perhaps with support) this should be sought. Considering the communication needs of the patient is of paramount importance in achieving a thorough assessment (C). It is essential to optimize your ability to communicate with the patient, and vice versa, by being aware of their communication needs. Communication difficulties may also be a significant contributing feature to their presenting complaint.

A collateral history (A) is of immense importance among patients with a learning disability, but should never take precedence over a patient's own history where possible.

While a formal MSE is desirable (B), it may not be possible or appropriate, particularly at a first appointment. Mental state can and should still be assessed but often needs to be modified according to the needs of the patient.

Developmental history (D) is an essential component of any learning disability new patient assessment.

Given the increased prevalence of physical co-morbidities in patients with learning difficulties, physical examination at new patient appointments (E) is more necessary than within general adult psychiatry setting.

However, consideration should be given to how, when, and by whom the physical assessment is best carried out.

→ Goldbart J, Caton S (2010). *Communication and People with the Most Complex Needs: What Works and Why This Is Essential*. Mencap, London.

5. E ★   OHPsych 3rd edn → p.736

In order to gain a detailed history about the change in functioning of this man, it is essential to ask for information from people who have regular contact with him, over a recent time period, and who are part of his day-to-day life. The residential home staff will be the best source as they care for him daily and will be aware of his functioning and the subsequent change (E). They are likely to have a lot of background information on him in their records and will keep daily written records which they can review.

His GP (A) will have good background medical and medication history but may lack the detail necessary to assess this presentation.

The man's girlfriend (B) is not his next of kin and she may not be able to provide an overview of his functioning in various domains. Given that he lives in a residential home, it is also possible that they do not live together, thus limiting the information she could give.

The medical ward staff (C) could give important information about his presentation on the ward but possibly little background history.

The man's parents (D) may be able to give a lot of information, but it is not clear whether they have a day-to-day role in his care.

→ Bradley E, Lofchy J (2005). Learning disability in the accident and emergency department. *Advances in Psychiatric Treatment*, **11**, 45–57.

6. A ★★   OHPsych 3rd edn → pp.730–1

Epilepsy occurs more commonly with increasing severity of learning disability across the range of causes of learning disability. Thus the answer is an IQ of < 20 (A).

WHO classification of learning disability is any IQ less than 70. It can be further subdivided as follows: profound learning disability: IQ of < 20; severe learning disability: IQ of 20–34 (B); moderate learning disability: IQ of 35–49 (C); and mild learning disability: IQ of 50–69 (D).

An IQ of 70 (E) falls within the normal range for IQ, albeit at the lower end of this range. Approximately 95% of the population scores between two standard deviations of the medium: between 70 and 130 points. IQ scores are derived from standardized tests to assess intelligence. The median score is 100 and the standard deviation is 15 points.

→ Epilepsy Society: http://www.epilepsysociety.org.uk/AboutEpilepsy/Epilepsyandyou/Epilepsyandlearningdisability-1.

7. B ★★   OHPsych 3rd edn → pp.742–3

Family therapy (B) is the most appropriate choice given the mention of complex attachment problems. This, as well as most forms of psychological therapy, is amenable to adaption to accommodate the potential specific needs of patients with learning disabilities.

Modified CBT (A) is commonly accessed by patients with learning disabilities. The work should be tailored to the patient's strengths and needs.

Narrative therapy (C) can be adapted for use with people with learning disabilities, although it is more commonly used in younger children. It is not seen as much as other therapies due partly to the limited number of trained narrative therapists. The process itself involves telling a 'story' of the problem, usually in an externalizing and playful manner, to help the therapist and patient explore problems.

There is no automatic restriction upon a person with a learning disability accessing any of the wide range of possible psychological therapy options. However, often the choice of therapy offered is a pragmatic mix of availability and suitability. IQ levels and cognitive abilities per se should not be considered solely as deciding factors (D).

Psychoanalytic psychotherapy (E) and its theoretical framework can be used where appropriate but would seldom be considered a first choice due to its demands.

→ RCPsych information on psychotherapy and learning disability: http://www.rcpsych.ac.uk/files/pdfversion/cr116.pdf.

→ Understanding Intellectual Disability and Health—Psychological Treatments for People with Learning Disabilities: http://www.intellectualdisability.info/mental-health/psychological-treatments-for-people-with-learning-disabilities.

8. A ★★★   OHPsych 3rd edn → pp.744–5

When prescribing for patients with a learning disability, the guiding principle is to 'start low and go slow' (A). While special consideration must always be given to concomitant medication and potential associated physical health problems, prescribing principles should be considered to be broadly similar to that for the general population once firm diagnoses have been made. Patients prescribed any medication should also be reviewed more frequently to titrate the dose up as required and monitor for side-effects.

Starting antidepressant at normal initiation dose and titrating up at normal titration rate (B) may be too rapid a titration regime and lead to unwanted side-effects.

Best practice would dictate up titrating the antidepressant more slowly, rather than more rapidly than usual (C).

Where practicable only one medication should be initiated at a time, so it would be better to start the antidepressant alone and titrate up as needed. Where used, benzodiazepines should be used at as low a dose and for as short a time as possible (D).

It is better to trial one medication at a time, so starting both an antidepressant and an antipsychotic together is best avoided (E).

→ RCPsych POMH UK information about medicines for people with learning disability: http://www.kmpt.nhs.uk/Downloads/Trust-Services/easy-read-information-people-ld.pdf.

Extended Matching Questions

1. A ★★

Short stature and low-set ears could be observed in a number of syndromes, for example Turner's syndrome (usually accompanied by a webbed neck and low hairline) and Noonan's syndrome (occurring in males and is accompanied by subnormal fertility.) Depression has a prevalence of around 10% in people with Down's syndrome.

2. E ★★

Again, all other features in this scenario could be suggestive of a number of syndromes; however, food-seeking is characteristic of a person with Prader–Willi syndrome as they are unable to feel satiated, with resultant central obesity.

3. B ★★

This scenario describes the characteristic facial phenotype of a person with fragile X. A person with fragile X is likely to have symptoms similar to ASD, if not a diagnosis of ASD.

4. D ★★

The scenario suggests absence of neonatal Guthrie (heel-prick) test and therefore failure to achieve an early diagnosis of phenylketonuria (PKU). This baby will be missing the enzyme phenylalanine hydroxylase, which breaks down phenylalanine found in protein-rich foods. Build-up of phenylalanine causes damage to the central nervous system. If diagnosed through the heel-prick test, treatment involves a diet extremely low in phenylalanine, and prognosis is very good.

5. I ★★

The first three features could be present in any person with a learning disability. However, the skin changes are more suggestive of a particular syndrome. In particular the large number of light brown patches on the skin describe numerous cafe au lait spots, which are suggestive of TS if more than six are present.

General feedback on 1–5: OHPsych 3rd edn → pp.744–55

6. J ★★★★

VCFS is associated with an elevated risk of psychotic illness. The age of onset varies between early adolescence and early adulthood, with most onsets occurring in the late teens and early 20s. The catechol-O-methyltransferase (COMT) gene is located on chromosome 22q11 and this is in the 1.5-megabase VCFS microdeletion region. Thus all individuals with this disorder have only one copy of this gene, suggesting that COMT may be a candidate gene for psychosis in VCFS.

7. B ★★★★

Down's syndrome is associated with an increased risk of depression compared with the general population.

8. F ★★★★

Lesch–Nyhan syndrome is associated with marked self-injurious behaviours. It is an X-linked recessive syndrome, due to a mutation in the gene that codes for an enzyme responsible for uric acid metabolism. Without this enzyme hyperuricaemia occurs.

9. H ★★★★

Prader–Willi syndrome is associated with an increased incidence of OCD. It has a incidence of between 1:10 000 and 1:20 000 and this is usually due to the deletion of paternally derived chromosomes.

10. D ★★★★

Fragile X syndrome is associated with an increased incidence of ASD. It is the genetic syndrome that is considered the most common single-gene cause of autism as well as inherited cause of mental retardation amongst boys. As well as mild to severe learning disability there are pathognomonic physical signs: elongated face, protruding ears, and macro-orchidism (extremely large testes).

General feedback on 6–10: OHPsych 3rd edn → pp.750–6

→ A.D.A.M.—Fetal alcohol syndrome: http://www.ncbi.nlm.nih.gov/pubmedhealth/PMH0001909.

→ Dykens EM, Leckman JF, Cassidy SB (1996). Obsessions and compulsions in Prader–Willi syndrome. *Journal of Child Psychology and Psychiatry*, **37** (8), 995–1002.

→ Genetics Home Reference—Lesch–Nyhan syndrome: http://www.ghr.nlm.nih.gov/condition/lesch-nyhan-syndrome.

→ National Coalition for Health Professional Education in Genetics—Fragile X syndrome: http://www.nchpeg.org/index.php?option=com_content&view=article&id=134&Itemid=18.

→ Strydom A (2003). Down's syndrome. *The Lancet*, **362** (9377), 80–1.

→ VCFS Educational Foundation Inc—Velo-cardio-facial syndrome: http://www.vcfsef.org/about_vcfs.php.

Substance misuse psychiatry

Greg Lydall and Kelly Clarke

Clinicians in all areas of medicine are likely to encounter people with substance misuse issues, so an understanding of the key issues is essential. Human beings have used intoxicating substances, such as alcohol, nicotine, cannabis, and heroin, for millennia. Motivations might include experimentation, pleasure, social enhancement, or for physical or psychological pain management. Some people who use these legal and illegal substances experience problems related to their use, including loss of control, adverse consequences, withdrawals or cravings, damaged end organs, risky behaviour, and premature death. Substance misuse impacts not only on individual physical and mental health but also upon families and wider society by increased healthcare, criminal justice, social services, and unemployment costs.

Drug and alcohol problems affect between 10% and 25% of the population each year, and up to 35% of people have ever used illicit drugs. Alcohol, an intoxicating sedative, is the most commonly used drug, with 25% of the UK population drinking above 'low-risk' limits. In England in 2010 there were an estimated 300 000 opiate, crack-cocaine, and injecting drug users, and only half were in treatment.

Substance misuse is commonly associated with physical and mental health co-morbidity. The prevalence of co-existing mental health and substance use problems (termed 'dual diagnosis') may affect between 30% and 70% of those presenting to healthcare and social care settings.

In general, four interrelationships in dual diagnosis are recognized:

• substance use leading to social problems and psychological symptoms not amounting to a diagnosis
• substance use leading to social dysfunction and secondary psychiatric and physical illness
• substance use exacerbating an existing mental or physical health problem and associated social functioning
• primary psychiatric illness precipitating substance misuse which may also be associated with physical illness and affect social ability.

Given the array of substance misuse problems, an individual treatment approach is essential and may involve psychological, pharmacological, and social intervention. An empathic, non-judgemental clinical approach is essential to engage people with substance misuse problems. Motivational interviewing is an evidence-based talking therapy to help people in denial about their problems make changes for themselves and avoids imposing change prematurely. Therapeutic approaches including Relapse Prevention, CBT, and Mindfulness can be used to help people remain abstinent once they have stopped using substances. Where thoughts and feelings have been chemically suppressed for a long time, learning to cope with these may be a key part of therapy.

The notion of 'recovery' from addiction has a number of features, including voluntary abstinence and sobriety. Newer definitions of addiction recovery do not include abstinence per se (because this may be unrealistic for some) but include meaningful engagement in treatment, improved quality of life, and citizenship.

Management of dual diagnosis is more complex. Generally, treatment (or at least stabilization) of the substance misuse is first required to enable assessment and management of psychiatric symptoms. In clinical reality this is not always possible and a more pragmatic approach is advised. For example, someone both alcohol dependent and psychotic may require both detoxification and antipsychotic medication concurrently.

Greg Lydall and Kelly Clarke

Single Best Answers

1. At 18 years old, Paul is admitted to the medical ward. Over the last six months Paul's world has revolved around his flatmates and friends who all drink heavily. Paul's flatmates often come to his flat for a morning cup of coffee. He often returns to his flat in the afternoon, drunk, without even knowing he is drunk and no longer carries on in his life of college. His recent knowledge of his alcohol level for the last 48 hours of drinking is at a particular problem. Which single step is...

A. Acute paracetamol and/or benzodiazepine intake
B. Chlordiazepoxide and thiamine for acute alcohol withdrawal changes in
C. Thiamine and intravenous glucose for acute alcohol withdrawal in
D. Intravenous glucose and intravenous thiamine and glucose for withdrawal with
   follow up
E. Fluid and electrolyte

2. A 24-year-old woman walks in complaining of low mood while intoxicated.
   You note that she is her CAGE screen often return. She is incoherent and
   unable to engage in full role for interaction. She score on the Alcohol Use
   Disorders Identification Test (AUDIT). What is the single most appropriate
   immediate response?

A. Advise her to engage in an alcohol
B. Reduce her blood alcohol, FBC and LFTs
C. Further intervention
D. Offer a brief intervention
E. Outpatient detoxification

3. A 45-year-old man presents to the emergency department accompanied by two
   colleagues. He is confused. His colleagues are worried and concerned and
   feel he is ataxic, and would like him to undergo a test. Which is the
   single most likely underlying cause of his condition?

A. Korsakoff's psychosis
B. Wernicke's encephalopathy
C. Oral manifestations
D. Delirium tremens
E. Confabulation

QUESTIONS

Single Best Answers

1. An 18-year-old man is admitted to a psychiatric ward. For the last two weeks he has felt people were following him and has overheard strangers talking about him. He has ideas of reference, vivid auditory hallucinations, but with no clouding of consciousness. His family report social withdrawal, unusual behaviour over the last year, and that he has recently dropped out of college. He reports smoking joints almost daily for the last 12 months. Which is the *single* most appropriate diagnosis? ★

A Acute schizophrenia-like psychotic disorder

B Mental and behavioural disorders due to cannabis: amnesic state

C Mental and behavioural disorders due to cannabis: psychotic disorder, schizophrenia like

D Mental and behavioural disorders due to cannabis: withdrawal with delirium

E Paranoid schizophrenia

2. A 23-year-old woman sustains a minor limb injury while intoxicated with alcohol. This is her third ED visit in a month. She is treated and is assessed as sober and safe for discharge. She scores 4 out of 16 on the Fast Alcohol Screening Test (FAST). Which is the *single* most appropriate initial management? ★

A Advise complete abstinence from alcohol

B Follow-up bloods, including FBC and LFTs

C Inpatient admission

D Offer a brief intervention

E Outpatient detoxification

3. A 24-year-old woman is dependent on heroin, confirmed by two positive urine drug screens. She wants help to stop injecting and 'sort her life out', and would like to have a 'clear head'. Which is the *single* most appropriate drug to prescribe? ★

A Injectable diamorphine

B Injectable methadone

C Oral buprenorphine

D Oral lofexidine

E Oral methadone

4. A 43-year-old man drinks four pints of lager every night. He has low mood with poor concentration, low energy levels, disturbed sleep, and poor appetite for one month. He denies suicidal ideation or intentions. He scores 4 out of 4 using the CAGE questionnaire, and has agreed to reduce, then stop his drinking. Which is the *single* most appropriate management option? ★

A Reassess mental state after four weeks of abstinence

B Refer for CBT

C Refer for motivational interviewing

D Start SSRI medication

E Start TCA medication

5. A 54-year-old man is found on the streets, drowsy and vomiting. He is unkempt with a strong odour of alcohol, is ataxic, verbally aggressive, and slurring his words. His temperature is 37.5°C, heart rate 96 bpm, and BP 115/87 mmHg. Which is the *single* most appropriate diagnosis to exclude? ★★

A Alcohol intoxication

B Alcohol withdrawal

C Aspiration pneumonia

D Head injury

E Psychotic episode

6. A 40-year-old man with heroin dependency is beginning to recognize that his IV drug use is problematic and starts to look at the pros and cons of continuing drugs. He says that he is most concerned about dangers of 'backtracking'. Which is the *single* most appropriate interpretation of his behaviour? ★★★

A Consuming heroin by heating it on foil and inhaling the fumes

B Falling into a short unrousable sleep having injected the heroin

C Melting down the heroin prior to injection

D Pulling one's own blood into the syringe, then reinjecting it

E Selling drugs to finance one's own drug dependency

7. A 56-year-old man is admitted to a substance misuse unit for alcohol detoxification. Thirty-six hours after his last drink he develops ataxia, nystagmus, ophthalmoplegia, memory impairment, agitation, and severe tremor. Which is the *single* most appropriate medication combination to prescribe? ★★★

A Acamprosate, chlordiazepoxide (reducing regime), oral B vitamins

B Acamprosate, chlordiazepoxide (reducing regime), parenteral B vitamins

C Chlordiazepoxide (reducing regime), disulfiram, parenteral B vitamins

D Chlordiazepoxide (reducing regime), haloperidol, oral B vitamins

E Diazepam (reducing regime), haloperidol, parenteral B vitamins

8. A 40-year-old man was an alcoholic and heroin addict. He has now completed an alcohol detox and is receiving methadone maintenance treatment. He has an established diagnosis of emotionally unstable PD, borderline type. He would like to continue with his methadone treatment and to reduce the risk of alcohol relapse; he is particularly concerned about alcohol cravings. Psychosocial intervention is initiated. Which is the *single* most appropriate medication to prescribe? ★★★★

A Acamprosate

B Disulfiram

C Fluoxetine

D Haloperidol

E Naltrexone

Extended Matching Questions

Substance-related effects

For each scenario below, choose the *single* most likely substance to cause these effects from the list of options. Each option may be used once, more than once, or not at all. ★

A Alcohol

B Cannabis

C Cocaine

D Gamma-hydroxybutyrate (GHB)

E Heroin

F Ketamine

G LSD

H Mephedrone

I MDMA

J Nicotine

1. An 18-year-old woman took an illicit drug at a dance party. She has clenched teeth and muscle cramps. She is visually hallucinating, and is overfamiliar and tactile with nursing staff. Her temperature is 38°C.

2. A 30-year-old man has chest pain which started an hour ago. He appears exhilarated, confident, and energetic but very irritable. He has a temperature of 37.6°C, heart rate 120 bpm, and BP 160/100 mmHg.

3. A 19-year-old man took a tablet. He describes visual hallucinations and feeling as if he can taste music.

4. A 60-year-old divorced man sustains a minor injury during a fight after work. He is emotionally labile, disinhibited, slurring his words, and uncoordinated.

5. A 27-year-old homeless man was found unresponsive in the street. He was drowsy, with pinpoint pupils and his respiratory rate was six breaths per minute. Naloxone was administered, resulting in rapid resolution of symptoms.

Street names for drugs

For each of the following scenarios describing street drug names, choose the *single* most appropriate chemical name from the list of options below. Each option may be used once, more than once, or not at all. ★★★

A Amyl nitrite

B Cannabis

C Cocaine

D Diacetylmorphine

E Freebase cocaine

F GHB

G Ketamine

H Methamphetamine

I MDMA

J Phencyclidine

6. A 27-year-old man appears intoxicated with a staggering, unsteady gait and slurred speech. His eyes are bloodshot. He denies drinking alcohol and says he was given some 'angel dust' by a friend.

7. A 22-year-old bought several vials of a substance which he was told would be an aphrodisiac. He thinks they were called 'poppers.' He took one and felt an instantaneous headrush but was left with a pounding headache.

8. A 19-year-old woman is pregnant and concerned that her baby will be born addicted to drugs. She has been using 'crack' for at least three months and does not feel she can stop.

9. A 31-year-old man has taken 'crystal meth'. He is hyperactive, sweaty, and breathing very fast. He says he feels great with loads of sexual energy although quickly becomes aggressive when questioned.

10. A 29-year-old woman was found unconscious and unresponsive by her neighbours. She has needle track marks visible on her arms. In her possession were found drug paraphernalia including a burned silver spoon and aluminium foil. Earlier that evening she was heard arguing with a man about a delivery of 'horse'.

ANSWERS

Single Best Answers

1. C ★ OHPsych 3rd edn → pp.62–3; 1026–8

The answer is mental and behavioural disorders due to cannabis: psychotic disorder, schizophrenia like (C). Drug-induced psychoses are characterized by a cluster of psychotic phenomena that occur during or immediately after psychoactive substance use and are characterized by vivid hallucinations (typically auditory, but often in more than one sensory modality), ideas of reference (often of a paranoid or persecutory nature), psychomotor disturbances, and other psychosis-like symptoms. The sensorium is usually clear, but some degree of clouding of consciousness may be present. While on the ward he should ideally have no access to illicit drugs (confirmed by repeat urine testing), and the symptoms should resolve at least partially within one month and fully within six months. Particular care should be taken to avoid diagnosing a more serious condition like schizophrenia when a diagnosis of drug-induced psychosis is more appropriate. A diagnosis of psychotic disorder should not be made merely on the basis of perceptual distortions or hallucinatory experiences when substances having primary hallucinogenic effects (e.g. LSD, mescaline, cannabis at high doses) have been taken.

In acute schizophrenia-like psychotic disorder the psychotic symptoms are comparatively stable and justify a diagnosis of schizophrenia but have lasted for less than about one month. The polymorphic unstable features (variable psychotic features and mood) are absent. If the schizophrenic symptoms persist for more than one month the diagnosis should be changed to schizophrenia. While the patient is using cannabis, as in this scenario, one cannot be certain that the psychotic features are not due to direct intoxication or drug induced. False diagnosis in such cases may have distressing and costly implications for the patient and for the health services (A).

Cannabis and alcohol can induce amnesia, but there is no mention of memory impairment in this case (B).

There is some debate on whether cannabis produces dependence and withdrawal. Either way there are no symptoms here to suggest a withdrawal state, including no evidence of physiological changes, or clouding of consciousness, which are typical in withdrawal states (D).

The diagnosis of schizophrenia is supported by the clinical symptoms (restricted affect, ideas of reference, vivid auditory hallucinations, psychomotor agitation) and possible prodromal symptoms (social withdrawal, unusual behaviour). However, he is still using cannabis, which complicates the picture, and the psychotic symptoms are short-lived (only two weeks). Many psychoactive substance-induced psychotic states are of short duration (e.g. amphetamine and cocaine psychoses). ICD-10 requires at least one month of either one of the FRSs, bizarre delusions, or two or more symptoms including persistent hallucinations, thought disorder, catatonic behaviour, negative symptoms, or significant and persistent behavioural change. ICD-10 recognizes that there may be a prodromal phase associated with schizophrenia, which is not included in the one-month time requirement (E).

→ ICD-10: http://www.who.int/substance_abuse/terminology/ICD10 ClinicalDiagnosis.pdf.

2. **D** ★   OHPsych 3rd edn → p.82

The most appropriate management is to offer a brief intervention (D). The FAST is a quick screening tool with a sensitivity of 93% and a specificity of 88% for detection of hazardous drinking (compared to the CAGE questionnaire with 40% and 98% respectively). The cut-off for clinical significance is 3/16 points on the FAST. By scoring 3+ the patient falls into the 'hazardous drinking' category at least. There is good evidence for 'screening and brief intervention' in an ED or primary care setting reducing hazardous drinking by 17% (NICE guideline on preventing alcohol use disorders). Brief alcohol interventions as short as five minutes have been shown to be effective in reducing alcohol consumption within primary care settings (Poikolainen, 1999; Wilk et al., 1997).

There is no evidence that recommending abstinence works (A), especially in this age group.

Follow-up bloods, including FBC and LFTs (B), are a good option to assess for alcohol-related damage, but not as important as the initial management option in this case (C). NICE do not recommend use of biochemical measures 'as a matter of routine' to screen for harmful or hazardous use.

There is no evidence that this woman is suffering from a mental or physical illness which would necessitate admission. Although admission is the 'safest' possible management it is not cost-effective or pragmatic in most instances (C).

The FAST does not detect alcohol dependence specifically. The CAGE is considered more useful for detecting severe alcohol dependence (with a cut-off of 2/4). In this case we do not know yet if the patient is alcohol dependent, and therefore detoxification may not be appropriate (E).

→ Health Development Agency—FAST manual: http://www.nice.org. uk/niceMedia/documents/manual_fastalcohol.pdf.

→ NICE Public Health Guidance24—Alcohol-use disorders: http:// www.nice.org.uk/nicemedia/live/13001/48984/48984.pdf.

→ Poikolainen K (1999). Effectiveness of brief interventions to reduce alcohol intake in primary health care populations: a meta-analysis. *Preventive Medicine*, **28** (5), 503–9.

→ Wilk AI, Jensen NM, Havighurst TC (1997). Meta-analysis of randomized control trials addressing brief interventions in heavy alcohol drinkers. *Journal of General Internal Medicine*, **12**, 274–83.

3. C ★   OHPsych 3rd edn → pp.598–9

Buprenorphine, an opioid receptor partial agonist, is licensed for the treatment of opiate dependency (C). Substitute opioid treatment reduces illicit opioid use, overdoses, criminal activity, and drug-related deaths. Due to its partial agonist properties, buprenorphine prevents opioid withdrawal and also blocks the effects of additional opioids, and so discourages drug use 'on top'. Unlike methadone, buprenorphine allows patients more of a clear head with less sedation.

Injectable diamorphine (heroin) (A) is a recognized treatment but is rarely used, and is certainly not first line. It is sometimes used for intractable opioid injecting, where first-line treatments have been unsuccessful and where the risks of ongoing illicit use (overdose, blood-borne viruses, death) outweigh the risks of prescribing injectable heroin. The Randomised Injectable Opiate Treatment Trial (RIOTT) found that treatment with supervised injectable heroin leads to significantly lower use of street heroin than does supervised injectable methadone or optimized oral methadone.

Methadone can also be injected (B) where oral methadone or buprenorphine are insufficient (for example, intractable injectors). However, like injectable diamorphine, it requires supervision, is resource intensive, and is not popular with patients.

Lofexidine (D) is a central alpha-adrenoreceptor agonist licensed for the treatment of opioid withdrawal. Lofexidine is given to relieve the symptoms associated with opioid withdrawal including chills, sweating, piloerection, stomach cramps, muscle pain, and rhinorrhoea. The patient is not specifically requesting a detoxification, and opioid substitute prescribing (methadone or buprenorphine) is therefore a better option.

There is good evidence of methadone's efficacy in opioid dependency syndrome, and methadone is commonly prescribed. Methadone is an opioid, usually taken orally in liquid form. Methadone reduces drug-related injecting, overdoses, deaths, and criminal activity. However, many patients find it sedating and that it takes the edge off their emotions. As this patient wanted a 'clear head', methadone would not be the best option (E).

→ King's College London—RIOTT trial: http://www.kcl.ac.uk/iop/depts/addictions/research/drugs/riott.aspx.

→ Department of Health—Drug misuse and dependence: UK guidelines on clinical management: http://www.nta.nhs.uk/uploads/clinical_guidelines_2007.pdf.

4. A ★   OHPsych 3rd edn → p.562

The most appropriate management option is to reassess mental state after four weeks of abstinence (A). When managing a patient who has both problem alcohol use and a co-morbid depressive disorder, the alcohol misuse should be treated initially as this may lead to improvement in their depressive symptoms. Furthermore, pharmacological and psychological treatments are unlikely to be effective in the presence of alcohol; these treatments should usually only be considered if depression continues after a period of abstinence from alcohol.

Psychological intervention is unlikely to be effective in the presence of continuing alcohol misuse. CBT (B) should be considered for people with symptoms of depression that persist after a period of abstinence from alcohol.

In this case, the patient appears motivated to stop drinking. Motivational interviewing (C) is a helpful treatment option for patients who are unable to reduce or stop their substance misuse. Using a non-confrontational empathic approach, the differences between the patient's personal ideals and their current behaviour are elicited. This creates cognitive dissonance and encourages the patient towards change. 'Change talk' is elicited and reinforced. The goal is to work with the patient towards positive change regarding their unhelpful behaviours.

Antidepressant therapy should only be considered after a period of abstinence from alcohol. If depressive symptoms continue, SSRIs (D), as the first-line choice of antidepressant, may be indicated. This patient is considered low risk of self-harm, and therefore more proactive treatment or referral to psychiatric services is not indicated at this time.

There is little evidence to support the efficacy of pharmacological treatment of depression in people who misuse alcohol and have a co-morbid depression disorder. If depression continues after a period of abstinence from alcohol, antidepressant treatment may be considered. TCAs (E) would not be the first-line choice of antidepressant in these circumstances due to their potential cardiotoxicity (especially in the context of alcohol misuse).

→ NICE Clinical Guideline 115—: http://www.nice.org.uk/guidance/CG115.

5. D ★★   OHPsych 3rd edn → pp.566–7

Head injury is the most important life-threatening complication of alcohol misuse that the doctor must exclude in this challenging but common scenario (D). Often head injuries have occurred but may not be reported by the patient.

Alcohol intoxication (A) might explain the clinical scenario—but it is unlikely to be life threatening unless there are physical co-morbidities or alcohol has been combined with other drugs.

Alcohol withdrawal (B) may explain the patient's odour of alcohol, unkempt appearance, and ataxia (the latter classically as part of Wernicke's syndrome), but in the absence of a tachycardia, sweating and tremor are unlikely.

Aspiration pneumonia (C) is not uncommon in heavy drinkers. The patient is afebrile, which makes the diagnosis of infection less likely (although not impossible).

Alcohol misuse and aggression are common in acute psychosis. However, in this scenario, organic causes need to be excluded first (E).

6. D ★★★   OHPsych 3rd edn → p.579

The answer is pulling one's own blood into the syringe, then reinjecting it is a means to ensure that none of the drug in the syringe is lost (D). It is thought by some users to be safe because it involves using one's own blood as the flush; however, if needles (or the syringe tube) are shared then there is a much greater risk of cross-contamination.

Consuming heroin by heating it on foil and inhaling the fumes (A) is called 'chasing' or 'chasing the dragon'. It is thought by some users to be safer than injection as it removes the risk of HIV and other blood-borne infections; however, it can expose the lungs to unfiltered pollutants.

Falling into a short unrousable sleep having injected the heroin (B) is called 'nodding' or 'gouching' and is subjectively a pleasant experience for the user but can leave the asleep user at risk of being robbed, attacked, or in danger from local environmental hazards.

Melting down the heroin prior to injection (C) is called 'cooking up' which is thought to sterilize the drugs by killing any bacteria in the drugs or the water (which could cause infection or abscesses). There are many dangers from this method including burns and open flames.

Selling drugs to finance one's own drug dependency (E) is called 'juggling'. It is commonly the manner whereby a drug user is able to maintain their lifestyle: by buying a larger amount of drug than is needed and reselling it to others (sometimes cut with a filler material to increase the weight). This can leave the seller at risk of police action, or criminal action, and fiscal risk. It adds to increased pressure to the drug user who now has to balance drug use and profits.

7. B ★★★   OHPsych 3rd edn → pp.560–1

Acamprosate is a GABA agonist and NMDA antagonist, licensed for treatment of alcohol dependence. Studies show that it reduces cravings, rates of relapse, and severity of relapse. Several studies support use in alcohol withdrawal because it is considered neuroprotective, with few side-effects or risks. Use of chlordiazepoxide and parenteral B vitamins is essential, and acamprosate probably helpful, making (B) the best answer.

This patient in alcohol withdrawal has the classic Wernecke's encephalopathy triad which usually presents 24–48 hours after the last drink. Treatment includes a reducing regime of either chlordiazepoxide or diazepam (to reduce CNS overexcitation) and high-potency parenteral (IM or IV) B vitamins. The oral vitamin route as in option (A) is incorrect due to impaired B vitamin absorption in these patients caused by alcoholic villous atrophy. The other medications are usually well absorbed.

Under normal metabolism, alcohol is broken down in the liver by the enzyme alcohol dehydrogenase to acetaldehyde, which is then converted by acetaldehyde dehydrogenase to acetic acid. Disulfiram (C) blocks the breakdown of acetaldehyde by antagonizing the enzyme acetaldehyde dehydrogenase. The resultant acetaldehyde build-up produces an unpleasant flushing reaction which may deter people from drinking. A severe reaction may cause cardiovascular instability; therefore it is used only in well-motivated patients. Its use in acute withdrawal is not supported mainly because if there is still alcohol in the patient's bloodstream they will experience an unpleasant, possibly even life-threatening, reaction.

Haloperidol (D), a typical antipsychotic, is often prescribed for acute psychosis or agitation. Haloperidol lowers seizure threshold and increases the risk of alcohol withdrawal seizures; therefore it is not typically used in alcohol withdrawal.

Diazepam (E) is a good alternative to chlordiazepoxide. However, use of haloperidol makes this an incorrect option.

8. A ★★★★   OHPsych 3rd edn → pp.564–5

There is good evidence of acamprosate's efficacy in preventing alcohol relapse (A). Acamprosate is a glutamatergic NMDA receptor antagonist; because alcohol dependence and alcohol withdrawal are associated with a hyperglutamatergic system, acamprosate effectively reduces this. According to NICE acamprosate should be prescribed as a first-line treatment with an individual psychosocial intervention. Furthermore, there is evidence that acamprosate reduces cravings whereas dilsulfiram, the only other viable option here, does not.

Disulfiram (B) is a good option to reduce risk of alcoholic relapse; however, acamprosate, in combination with a psychosocial intervention, is recommended by NICE as first-line therapy for maintenance of abstinence from alcohol. Disulfiram is contraindicated in people with severe PD because of the risk of impulsive drinking on top of disulfiram which could lead to cardiovascular instability and even death.

There is no strong evidence that treatment with an SSRI (C) or antipsychotic (D) is effective in reducing alcoholic relapse.

Naltrexone (E) was licensed in 2012 in the UK for maintenance of abstinence in alcohol dependence syndrome. However, it is contraindicated here due to its mu-opioid receptor antagonist properties, which in this patient on methadone maintenance would precipitate acute opioid withdrawal. Therefore, patients using opioids or requiring opioid-based analgesia should not be treated with naltrexone.

→ NICE Clinical Guideline 115—Alcohol dependence and harmful alcohol use: http://guidance.nice.org.uk/CG115/NICEGuidance/pdf/English.

Extended Matching Questions

1. I ★

Classic MDMA effects are: mild hallucinogenic effects; increased tactile sensitivity; empathic feelings; teeth clenching; muscle cramping; sleep disturbances; depression; hyperthermia; addiction.

2. C ★

This describes stimulant effects. Cocaine is classically known to cause increased heart rate, BP, and body temperature; feelings of exhilaration; increased energy; reduced appetite; irritability; anxiety; paranoia; violent behaviour; psychosis; weight loss; insomnia; myocardial infarction; stroke; seizures; addiction.

3. G ★

Synaesthesia (stimulation of one sensory or cognitive pathway leads to automatic, involuntary experiences in a second sensory or cognitive pathway) is the giveaway effect of LSD which is not described with any of the others (cannabis would fit with the rest of the descriptions). LSD also causes altered states of perception and feeling; hallucinations; sleeplessness; dizziness; weakness.

4. A ★

This classic alcohol intoxication picture does not fit with any of the other options (including nicotine and GHB—these do not directly cause neurologic deficits, hypertension, or heart disease). Alcohol's effects also include: euphoria; relaxation; lowered inhibitions; drowsiness; slurred speech; emotional volatility; loss of coordination; impaired memory; loss of consciousness; increased risk of injuries or violence; depression; addiction; fatal overdose.

5. E ★

Opioid effects include: euphoria; drowsiness; impaired coordination; dizziness; confusion; nausea; sedation; slowed or arrested breathing; constipation; endocarditis; addiction; fatal overdose. Giveaways in this scenario are endocarditis (from IV use), respiratory suppression, and pinpoint pupils.

General feedback on 1–5: OHPsych 3rd edn → pp.582–90

6. J ★★★

Phencyclidine is also known as PCP, or rocket fuel in its liquid form. Its psychological effects include hallucination and euphoria, but it can also cause suicidal impulses, paranoia, and aggression. Phencyclidine tends to alter mood states in an unpredictable fashion; some people become very lively while others experience depersonalization. A mixture of marijuana and phencyclidine is known as happy sticks.

7. A ★★★

Amyl nitrite (also known as alkyl nitrite) is inhaled to give the immediate effects of light-headedness and heightened senses which quickly fade after a few minutes. Aspirating the liquid can lead to lipoid pneumonia and ingesting it can cause cyanosis. If spilled on the skin it can cause chemical burns.

8. E ★★★

Crack is freebase cocaine which can be smoked for a short, intense high. It is considered to be more addictive than cocaine due to the desire to recapture the early experiences, which are more prolonged euphoria without the same comedown effects. Cocaine, known by many names including coke, crank, and snow, tends to be rubbed into the gums or snorted. Crack and phencyclidine is known as missile basing.

9. H ★★★

Methamphetamine is also known as crystal or ice. Side-effects include skin picking, priapism, and 'meth mouth', a dental condition characterized by severe loss of teeth, thought to be due to drug-induced teeth grinding combined with a dry mouth. Confusingly, heroin mixed with cocaine is called a speedball whereas (meth)amphetamines are more generally known as speed.

10. D ★★★

Diacetylmorphine is known more commonly by its original trade name of heroin and more colloquially as H, skag, smack, or brown. It is used for its intense relaxation and euphoria-producing qualities, which unfortunately quickly lead to tolerance, increased dependence, and withdrawal effects. The main adverse effects come from contaminants when diacetylmorphine is cut with other substances to increase its weight and from the methods used to take the drug, most often injection.

General feedback on 6–10: OHPsych 3rd edn → p.578

→ Comprehensive list of illicit drug and street names (American website): http://www.drugrehab.co.uk/street-drug-names.htm.

Chapter 13

Liaison psychiatry and organic illness

Andrew Horton and Mark Broadhurst

Liaison psychiatry is a subspecialty of psychiatry which involves the diagnosis, treatment, and management of psychiatric illness in patients who have physical illnesses or present with physical symptoms.

There is considerable overlap between psychiatric and medical conditions which requires close working relationships with medical colleagues. Liaison psychiatry is a fascinating area where the range of psychiatric presentations is wide, every case is different, and there is opportunity to keep up to date with medicine as it evolves.

Within the UK there are different models practiced in different areas, ranging from assessment and signposting services to services with provision for long-term outpatient follow-up. There is increasing interest in the provision of liaison services in primary care because of the challenges faced by GPs in treating patients with medically unexplained symptoms. Another driver is the hugely increased morbidity and mortality rates seen in patients with co-morbid physical and mental illnesses who receive the majority of their treatment in secondary care.

Andrew Horton and Mark Broadhurst

QUESTIONS

Single Best Answers

1. A 56-year-old man is admitted to the surgical unit following a routine hernia operation. The nursing staff are concerned that he may be suffering from post-operative delirium. Which *single* feature is characteristic of this diagnosis? ★

A Clouding of consciousness

B Gradual stepwise onset

C Nihilistic delusions

D Normal sleep–wake cycle

E Orientation to time

2. A 22-year-old scaffolder has a head injury following a fall. His partner asks about the likelihood of personality changes or cognitive impairment following this head injury. Which *single* factor is the most likely to increase the chance of these sequelae? ★

A Dominant hemisphere involvement

B Evidence of leukoariosis

C Post-traumatic amnesia of four hours

D Unilateral hemisphere involvement

E Younger age

3. A 31-year-old teacher is reviewed in the outpatient clinic. He has discussed his suicidal thoughts with his wife. Which *single* feature is a risk factor for completed suicide? ★

A Discussion about suicide with relative

B Employment status

C Male gender

D Marriage status

E Young age

4. A 27-year-old man is diagnosed with a meningioma of the frontal lobe. His partner asks about clinical symptoms related to frontal lobe syndrome. Which is the *single* most likely feature of this? ★

A Auditory hallucinations

B Persecutory delusions

C Poor judgement

D Pressure of speech

E Thought disorder

5. A 62-year-old woman with schizoaffective disorder requires an angiogram following a myocardial infarction. There is concern regarding her capacity to consent for this. She is able to understand, weigh up the information, and communicate her decision. Which *single* additional factor is required to make a decision under the Mental Capacity Act? ★

A Agree with the information

B Listen to the information

C Retain the information

D Take the advice of her doctor

E Write down the information

6. A 22-year-old man has HIV. His partner has read about HIV and the increased risk of mental health problems. He would like to know the commonest mental health disorder to look out for. Which is the *single* most appropriate answer? ★★

A Delirium

B Dementia

C Depression

D Mania

E Psychosis

7. A 19-year-old man experiences an unusual sensation in his stomach. Although he becomes drowsy, he does not lose consciousness. There is a strong sense of familiarity which he has difficulty describing after the event. Which *single* type of seizure best describes these symptoms? ★★

A Absence seizure

B Complex partial seizure

C Generalized tonic-clonic seizure

D Myoclonic seizure

E Simple partial seizure

8. A 42-year-old woman is admitted to a medical ward with abdominal discomfort, confusion, and pain in her legs. She describes drowsiness, frequent urination, constipation, reduced motivation, and weight loss. Which is the *single* most likely underlying cause? ★★★

A Hypercalcaemia

B Hypernatraemia

C Hyperthyroidism

D Hypoglycaemia

E Hypokalaemia

Extended Matching Questions

Neurological diagnoses

For each scenario, choose the *single* most likely diagnosis from the list of options. Each option may be used once, more than once, or not at all. ★

A Acute intermittent porphyria

B Addison's disease

C Chronic subdural haematoma

D Creutzfeldt–Jakob disease

E HIV dementia

F Huntington's disease

G Multiple sclerosis

H Neurosyphilis

I Parkinson's disease

J Wilson's disease

1. A 58-year-old man has elevated mood, grandiose delusions, and is sexually disinhibited which is out of character. His wife reports that his memory has got worse in recent months and that he has difficulty walking. On further questioning he describes having an 'abnormality' on his penis some years ago.

2. A 41–year-old man has become more clumsy, with an increase in anxiety and memory problems. His wife describes that he often slurs his speech. He recalls that his father had unusual movements at a similar age.

3. A 70-year-old woman is referred to the outpatient clinic with depression. She has stiffness in her joints and a tremor at rest. She holds her elbows flexed, has difficulty starting to walk, and can only take small steps.

4. A 66-year-old woman with alcohol dependence is admitted to hospital. She appears drowsy with a delay in answering questions. Her friend reports concerns that she has been less alert and quite forgetful recently. She attended the ED a month ago to have a wound on her head sutured.

5. A 19-year-old student is unable to undertake his studies due to frequent mood disturbances. He finds it difficult to write due to a tremor and recently has had difficulty swallowing solid food. There is a green and brownish tinge to his cornea.

Medically unexplained symptoms

For each scenario below, choose the *single* most likely diagnosis from the list of options. Each option may be used once, more than once, or not at all. ★

A Adjustment disorder

B Body dysmorphic disorder

C Chronic fatigue syndrome

D Dissociative disorder

E Factitious disorder

F Generalized anxiety disorder

G Hypochondriasis

H Münchausen's by proxy

I Somatization disorder

J Somatoform pain disorder

6. A 40-year-old man thinks that his nose is abnormally large and asks his GP for a referral to a plastic surgeon so that this can be reduced. His family and friends do not think that there is anything wrong with his nose. He is too preoccupied with his appearance to go to work and stays indoors during the day.

7. A 34-year-old woman describes being 'unwell' since childhood. She has regular appointments with her GP with a variety of symptoms connected with her gastrointestinal system, skin, and menstrual periods. She also has visited several different EDs and has undergone several medical investigations. On each occasion, no underlying medical cause could be found.

8. A 52-year-old man, whose father has recently died of a stroke, develops paralysis in his right arm. Physical examination does not reveal a pattern of motor or sensory loss that is consistent with an underlying pathology.

9. A 29-year-old man comes to the ED with a urine sample. Testing reveals blood in his urine. He is admitted to hospital, but no further abnormality is found on urine testing. When challenged, he discharges himself from hospital.

10. A 62-year-old man is concerned that he has bowel cancer. Although he has lost weight recently this is explained by an increase in exercise. He believes that his stools are darker and this is a sign of cancer. Despite undergoing numerous tests with normal results and reassurance from several doctors he still believes he has cancer.

ANSWERS

Single Best Answers

1. A ★   OHPsych 3rd edn → pp.790–2

Delirium is extremely common on medical and surgical wards (10–20%). Clouding of consciousness is commonly found (A).

The onset of clinical features in delirium is often rapid rather than gradual (B). Gradual stepwise onset of symptoms is a feature of vascular dementia.

Paranoid delusions as opposed to nihilistic delusions (C) are seen in the delirious patient.

Delirium usually involves disturbance of the sleep–wake cycle (D). Other clinical features include global impairment of cognition, impairment of recent memory, perceptual disturbance (illusions and hallucinations), and incoherent speech.

Disorientation in time (E) is common in delirious patients.

→ Sanders RD, Pandharipande PP, Davidson AJ, Ma D, Maze M (2011). Anticipating and managing post-operative delirium and cognitive decline in adults. *British Medical Journal*, **343**, d4331.

2. A ★   OHPsych 3rd edn → pp.154–5

Dominant hemisphere involvement (A) is associated with an increased risk of psychiatric morbidity.

Leukoariosis is not the correct answer (B). It describes non-specific changes seen in white matter on brain imaging. Its presence post-head injury is not associated with increased psychiatric morbidity.

An increased duration of post-traumatic amnesia increases risk (C), as opposed to this short duration of four hours.

Bilateral hemisphere rather than unilateral involvement (D) is associated with increased risk.

Head injury is common, with a peak incident between the ages of 15 and 24 years old. However, older age rather than younger age (E) is associated with an increased risk of psychiatric morbidity.

→ Brooks DN, McKinlay W (1983). Personality and behavioural change after severe blunt head injury—a relative's view. *Journal of Neurology, Neurosurgery and Psychiatry*, **46** (4), 336–44.

3. C ★   OHPsych 3rd edn → pp.784–5

Males (C) are a higher risk of completed suicide when compared to females. Any mental disorder (greatest risk in major depression and anorexia) and dependence on alcohol or drugs also increase the risk.

Discussion of his suicidal thoughts with his wife does not increase his risk of completed suicide (A).

Employment status is associated with suicide risk, in that unemployment and retirement both increase risk (B). Therefore the patient's occupation as a teacher is not a factor that increases his risk of suicide.

Living alone and being single, divorced, or widowed are risk factors, rather than being married (D).

Older age increases the risk of suicide and it is estimated that 20% of all suicides are of the elderly (E).

→ Borges G, Nock MK, Haro Abad JM, et al. (2010). Twelve-month prevalence of and risk factors for suicide attempts in the World Health Organization World Mental Health Surveys. *Journal of Clinical Psychiatry*, **71** (12), 1617–28.

4. C ★   OHPsych 3rd edn → pp.72–3

Frontal lobe syndrome may be caused by a range of diseases (e.g. cerebrovascular, degenerative) or head trauma. Patients may present with poor judgement (C), euphoric mood, sexual disinhibition, or a change in personality.

Auditory hallucinations (A) are associated with psychotic illnesses, and are an FRS of schizophrenia.

Persecutory delusions (B) are associated with psychotic illnesses and are the most common type of delusions in schizophrenia.

Pressure of speech (D) can be a feature of mania, not frontal lobe syndrome.

Frontal lobe syndrome leads to cognitive difficulties such as short attention span, poor memory, and difficulty planning and reasoning. Thought disorder (E) is not typically seen as part of frontal lobe syndrome.

→ David A, Fleminger S, Kopelman MD, Lovestone S, Mellers JDC (2012). *Lishman's Organic Psychiatry. A Textbook of Neuropsychiatry*, 4th edn. Wiley-Blackwell, Oxford, pp.58–60.

5. C ★   OHPsych 3rd edn → pp.794–5

It is important to be aware of how to assess capacity for specific decisions. When assessing capacity the patient must be able to understand the information relevant to the decision, use or weigh up the information, retain the information (C), and communicate the decision.

Although patients are required to weigh up information given relating to a capacity decision, this is not the same as a requirement to agree with or believe the information given (A).

Patients usually need to listen to information (B) in order to fulfill the other aspects of the capacity assessment, but this is not required. For example, information may be relayed to hard-of-hearing patients by sign language, lip reading, or giving written information.

Respect for the autonomy of competent patients (patients with capacity) means patients can make decisions considered unwise by doctors. Competent patients do not have to take clinicians' advice, even if their decision may lead to their death (D).

Writing down information (E) may help competent patients make decisions, and may facilitate capacity assessments. It is not a legal requirement of the Mental Capacity Act.

→ National Archives—Mental Capacity Act (2005): http://www.legislation.gov.uk/ukpga/2005/9/contents.

6. C ★★ OHPsych 3rd edn → pp.162–3

Thirty to fifty percent of individuals with HIV will suffer from depression (C).

Delirium (A) occurs in approximately 30% of infected patients. This may be caused by direct infection of the brain or by secondary infections of tumours.

HIV-associated dementia (B) is a relatively common outcome in AIDS not HIV.

Manic symptoms (D) may occur as a result of the illness or due to the medication (antiretrovirals) prescribed, but are not as common as depressive symptoms.

Atypical, bizarre psychotic symptoms (E) are less likely to occur in the context of HIV infection.

→ WHO report: HIV/AIDS and mental health (2008): http://apps.who.int/gb/ebwha/pdf_files/EB124/B124_6-en.pdf.

7. B ★★ OHCM, 9th edn → pp.378–81

An altered awareness of self and environment is experienced in complex partial seizures (B). Seizures originating in the temporal lobe can give rise to an aura which in this case is the unusual sensation in this man's stomach. Auras can occur in any modality. Déjà vu (intense sense of familiarity) can also be experienced. Consciousness is generally not lost, but the altered awareness may lead to a range of psychiatric features.

In absence attacks (A), the patient has a sudden loss of awareness which lasts for seconds and ends abruptly. Simple automatisms may occur such as eye blinking. Absence seizures generally present in childhood.

Generalized tonic-clonic seizures (C) are of sudden onset where the limbs stiffen (tonic) and then jerk (clonic). After the convulsion the patient may present as unrousable, sleepy, or disorientated for some time. Other associated features may include incontinence, tongue biting, or other injuries.

The patient may experience sudden, brief, involuntary muscle contraction in myoclonic seizures (D).

In simple partial seizures (E), consciousness is not impaired and the content depends on the site of the focus. Focal neurological or cognitive dysfunction may persist.

→ Gelder M, Harrison P, Cowen P (2006). *Shorter Oxford Textbook of Psychiatry*, 5th edn. Oxford University Press, Oxford, pp.346–50.

→ Longmore M, Wilkinson I, Davidson E, Foulkes A, Mafi A (2004). *Oxford Handbook of Clinical Medicine*, 8th edn. Oxford University Press, Oxford, pp.378–81.

8. A ★★★ OHCM, 9th edn → pp.692

Hypercalcaemia (A) causes symptoms that are summarized by the mnemonic: bones, stones, groans, and psychic moans. Gastrointestinal symptoms include abdominal pain, vomiting, constipation, and weight loss. Urinary symptoms include polyuria, renal stones, and renal failure. Bone pain and drowsiness may occur. Hypercalcaemia can often present with psychiatric symptoms (depression, anorexia, confusion).

Raised sodium (hypernatraemia) (B) may be caused by an increase in water loss in excess of sodium. This may be caused by drugs, e.g. carbamazepine. The patient may appear dehydrated (dry skin, reduced skin turgor, postural hypotension) with confusion and seizures.

Symptoms of hyperthyroidism (C) include weight loss, increased appetite, diarrhoea, sweating, and tremor. The patient may appear irritable with psychotic features.

Decreased blood glucose (hypoglycaemia) (D) may present in a fashion similar to psychiatric disorders. The patient may present with personality change, mannerisms, restlessness, and mutism. There is often a change in consciousness, with the patient appearing drowsy.

Hypokalaemia (E) can cause abnormalities in the ECG, including small/inverted T-wave, prolonged P-R interval, and depressed ST segment. Signs of decreased potassium include muscle weakness, hypotonia, and cardiac arrhythmias.

→ Longmore M, Wilkinson I, Davidson E, Foulkes A, Mafi A (2004). *Oxford Handbook of Clinical Medicine*, 8th edn. Oxford University Press, Oxford, p.692.

Extended Matching Questions

1. H ★

Neurosyphilis is caused by a spirochaete infection of the brain. It usually manifests in males in their 40s and 50s, roughly 15–20 years after initial infection. The abnormality on his penis suggests primary infection with syphilis which can present as a painless lesion. Psychiatric symptoms can include grandiosity, euphoria, and mania, with mood-congruent delusions. There may also be disinhibition, personality change, and memory impairment.

2. F ★

Huntington's disease is a genetic disease characterized by a progressive dementia and worsening chorea. The disease has autosomal dominant inheritance. Features include chorea, dementia, and a family history of Huntington's disease. The choreiform movements are involuntary and include tics, jerks, grimacing, and dysarthria. There is increased tone with rigidity and stiffness. Depression and anxiety are common, with psychosis occurring early in the disease.

3. I ★

Parkinson's disease typically has its onset in the 50s and peaks during the 70s, with males affected more frequently than females. Depression is common (40–70%). Psychosis also occurs, and may be due to the medication prescribed. Clinical features include: a 'pill rolling' tremor which increases with anxiety or fatigue and diminishes during sleep; rigidity, often called 'lead pipe' or 'cogwheel rigidity'; bradykinesia, seen as slowness of initiating movements, reduced facial expression, and blinking; a 'festinant gait' with reduced arm swing and other postural abnormalities and autonomic instability.

4. C ★

Chronic subdural haematomas may manifest after months with no suggestion of recent trauma. In this case the prior head wound suggests that the patient may have suffered a fall. Headache, altered level consciousness, and amnesia may occur. The mental state may be variable on different occasions, with periods of unusual drowsiness.

5. J ★

Wilson's disease is a rare genetic disorder that involves an abnormality of copper metabolism. Copper deposits in the liver cause cirrhosis and in the basal ganglia cause neurological signs. Psychiatric symptoms may also occur, particularly mood disturbance, psychosis, and dementia. Onset is usually in childhood or early adulthood. Extrapyramidal signs include tremor, dystonia, and bulbar signs. Kayser–Fleisher rings (green-brown corneal deposits) are the ocular abnormality in this case.

General feedback on 1–5: OHPsych 3rd edn. → pp.133, 168–72

6. B ★

In body dysmorphic disorder patients have a preoccupation that an aspect of their body is abnormal or unattractive. This preoccupation causes significant distress and is considered an overvalued idea. As a result, those affected may seek surgical procedures. The most commonly affected areas include the face, head, and sexual organs.

7. I ★

Somatization disorder is where there are repeated presentations with medically unexplained symptoms. These symptoms affect multiple organ systems, with discrepancy between objective and subjective findings. They can be focused on one system but may move to a different system once exhaustively investigated and found to be negative. The sites of the body commonly affected include the gastrointestinal system, skin, and sexual and gynaecological functions.

8. D ★

Dissociative disorder occurs usually as a result of a severe psychological stressor with which the patient is unable to cope. Initially it may appear that there is an underlying physical cause, but following examination that does confirm any underlying pathology a psychological cause is identified. The symptoms are not produced intentionally and secondary gain is not part of this diagnosis.

9. E ★

In factitious disorder the patient intentionally fabricates signs of physical or mental illness. These can mimic any physical or mental illness, with behaviours including self-induced infections, self-medication, and altering records.

10. G ★

Hypochondriasis is the preoccupation of having a serious underlying medical illness despite negative investigations and reassurance. The underlying illness is often one that may lead to death or serious disability. The patient will often ruminate on normal variation of bodily functions. They may seek medical advice and investigation and fail to be reassured.

General feedback on 6–10: OHPsych 3rd edn → pp.796–814

Index

Note: Answers to questions appear in *italics*